# Acknowledgments

Thank you to my children, my sons Arūnas, Vidas, and my daughter Jolanta, for their continuous love and support.

I thank my husband Terry for his love and support.

Special thanks to my granddaughter Deimantė, who gave generosity of her time to illustrate and design my book.

This project could not have been accomplished without the support, guidance, and influence of many people. Much gratitude goes to the following key individuals: Joshua Rosenthal, founder and director of Institute for Integrative Nutrition for the health coach training program; Deborah King, master healer and teacher, who changed my life; My friend Lois Stevenson, teacher, for her editorial and review work throughout the writing process.

I thank Gretchen V. Fleming, for all the help with editing.

I thank Donna Marton, Kathy Davidson, Lindalee Stuckey, Nancy Rogers for reviewing and sharing their word of advice. I also want to thank my neighbor Peggy L. Bowes, a teacher and a researcher, for all the advices.

# CHOICES FOR
# HEALTHY
# LIVING

RAMUTE MOYE PhD

ISBN 979-8-88685-870-9 (paperback)
ISBN 979-8-88685-871-6 (digital)

Christian Faith Publishing
832 Park Avenue
Meadville, PA 16335
www.christianfaithpublishing.com

Illustrator and layout designer: Deimanté Gudelyté

Printed in the United States of America

# Contents

# Word from the Author

I was raised in Lithuania, a small country near the Baltic Sea. While growing up at the end of World War II, like so many other people at the time, my family had little food, which is why making a living was very difficult. Many days I went to school without bringing any lunch, and often one piece of bread was all the food I ate during the day. I began to think of ways to help to make life better for everyone in our country.

After watching how hard people at the time had to work to get food on the table, I wanted to become an agronomist. In my studies at the University of Agriculture in Lithuania, I learned how to develop technology for improving soil to increase agricultural production. At the time, farmers were encouraged to use a long list of chemicals to protect plants from disease and insects.

While working as a scientist at the Institute of Horticulture, my program was based on organic gardening. This program changed my life. I realized that the food we eat must be free from chemicals.

Over the last twenty years in the United States, I have been educated as a natural health consultant and became an energy healer and certified health coach. I believe that nutrition, lifestyle, clean water and environment and spirituality are the path to good health. I have resolved to use my life experience and education to help other people reach their goals, have good relationships, and enjoy life. I want to help others understand that they are more powerful than any circumstance they could encounter.

*I wish you a happy reading, and I hope I can help you find what you are looking for!*

*Ramute Moye*

## Chapter 1

# What's Your Risk?

One hundred years ago, very few Americans suffered from coronary heart disease, stroke, and cancer. Today these lifestyle-related illnesses account for the majority of deaths in America. The facts show that heart disease is the leading cause of death for both men and women.

## Health Risks

Heart disease

About 630,000 Americans die from heart disease each year; that's one in every four deaths. Coronary heart disease is the most common type of heart disease, killing about 366,000 people in 2015. In the United States, someone has a heart attack every forty seconds. Heart diseases cost the United States about $200 billion each year. This total includes the cost of health-care services, medications, and lost productivity.

Diabetes

Diabetes dramatically increased in the last decade. In the USA, there are more than thirty million people with diabetes. Diabetes is the leading cause of blindness, kidney failure, and amputations. Living with diabetes places an enormous emotional, physical, and financial burden on the entire family. Annually, diabetes costs the American public more than $245 billion.

Obesity

The National Center for Health Statistics shows more than one in three adults (37.7%) were considered to have obesity. Obesity has become a serious health problem in the United States.

What *is the impact of obesity on society?* Obesity has taken a toll on health-care costs across the country, estimating between $147 billion and $210 billion in direct and indirect health-care costs as of 2010. Lifetime medical costs for a ten-year-old child with obesity are staggering, about $19,000 more per child when compared with a child of healthy weight. When multiplied by the number of ten-year-old children with obesity in America, lifetime health-care expenses are estimated to be $14 billion. Obesity is considered an unhealthy body and mind. It can increase the risk of developing chronic health problems (stroke, heart disease, diabetes, etc.).

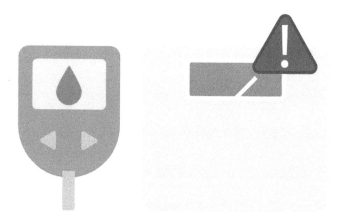

Cancer

*Cancer statistics by the National Cancer Institute United States.* Cancer statistics describe what happens in large groups of people who are diagnosed with and die from cancer each year and the number of people who are still alive at a given time after diagnosis people died from the disease. Each year, more than half a million Americans, which is more than 1,500 people a day, die of cancer.

Estimated national expenditures for cancer care in the United States in 2017 were $147.3 billion. In future years, costs are likely to increase as the population ages, and cancer prevalence increases. We know how hard it is on us since most cancer types cause death.

Food sensitivities and allergies

The body's immune system is meant to identify and destroy germs (such as bacteria or viruses) that make us sick. However, our absorptive ability is severely restricted when the lining of our intestines becomes irritated or flattened. This can occur with food allergies, food intolerances, and/or inflammatory bowel diseases. If these issues aren't resolved, nutrient absorption will not occur.

*What is food intolerance?* Symptoms of food intolerance are milder and usually have a slower onset than food allergy (but not always). These symptoms can include gas/bloating, diarrhea, stomach cramping, stuffy nose, mucus production, nausea, vomiting, headaches, etc. Common culprits are wheat, milk, corn, and more recently, soy. Lactose intolerance is a common example.

*How you may prevent food sensitivities.*

- Varying the diet
- Avoiding high quantities of high risk foods
- Getting breastfed for the first year of life
- Limiting excessive amounts of caffeine
- Avoiding compounds that increase gut permeability, such as alcohol, spicy foods, raw pineapple, raw papaya, aspirin, and other nonsteroidal anti-inflammatory drugs (NSAIDs)
- Limiting exposure to pesticides, herbicides, and fungicides used on food crops

If you suspect you may have food sensitivity, it's important to first rule out the possibility of a true food allergy. This can be done with your physician. If you suspect you may have a food intolerance, keeping a diligent food diary/response log can help you find the offending foods quickly and remove them.

*What is a food allergy?* An allergic reaction to food involves an immune system response that starts with a protein molecule made by the body, called an antibody, which helps battle viruses and bacteria. An antibody can connect with and attach to a specific target, known as its antigen, which is usually located on the virus, bacterium, or allergen. Once bound to the invader, it's like a red alert, calling out the invading allergen, and provoking the body's immune system to attack it.

*Food allergens.* The eight most common food allergens:

- Milk
- Eggs
- Peanuts
- Tree nuts (e.g., almonds, cashews, walnuts)
- Fish
- Shellfish
- Soy
- Wheat

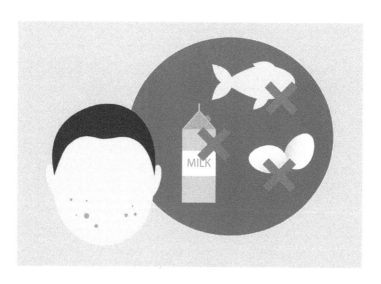

It's estimated that 3–7% of children and about 2% of adults suffer from food allergy.

## What Problems Must Be Solved?

Health and environment

Health is wholeness. It is a concept that cannot apply solely to an individual, since people and other beings have always lived within families, communities, ecosystems, and planetary-level conditions. The health of any part of the whole of this nested set of relationships is dependent on diverse, dynamic interaction among them all.

*Major environmental problems:*

1. *Pollution*: pollution of air, water, and soil require clean up. Industry and motor vehicle exhaust are the number one pollutants. Heavy metals, nitrates, and plastic are toxins responsible for pollution. While water pollution is caused by oil spills and urban runoff, air pollution is caused by various gases and toxins released by industries and factories and combustion of fossil fuels. The majority of soil pollution is caused by industries' waste that deprives soil of essential nutrients.
2. *Waste disposal:* Plastic, fast-food packaging and cheap electronic wastes threaten the well-being of humans. Waste disposal is an urgent current environmental problem.
3. *Loss of biodiversity:* Human activity is leading to the extinction of species and habitats and loss of biodiversity. Ecosystems, which took millions of years to perfect, are in danger when any species' population is decimating. A balance of natural processes, like pollination, is crucial to the survival of the ecosystem. One example is the destruction of coral reefs in the various oceans, which support the rich marine life.

4. *Water pollution*: Clean drinking water is becoming a rare commodity. Water is becoming an economic and political issue as human populations fight for this resource. One of the options suggested is using the process of desalinization. Industrial development is filling our rivers, seas, and oceans with toxic pollutants which are a major threat to human health.

5. *Urban sprawl*: Urban sprawl refers to migration of population from high density urban areas to low density rural areas. This results in spreading cities over more and more rural land. Urban sprawl brings land degradation, increased traffic, environmental issues, and health issues. The current environmental problems pose a lot of risk to the health of humans and animals. Dirty water is the biggest health risk to the quality of life and health.

Addiction and health

Addiction is a brain disorder and physical inability to stop consuming a chemical, drug, activity, or substance. Drug use can also increase the risk of contracting infections. Some people with disorders like anxiety or depression may use drugs in an attempt to alleviate psychiatric symptoms, which may exacerbate their mental disorder in the long run, as well as increase the risk of developing addiction.

Drug use increases the spread of infectious diseases. Injection of drugs accounts for one in ten cases of HIV. Injection drug use is also a major factor in the spread of hepatitis C and can be the cause of endocarditis and cellulitis. Drugs that are misused can cause intoxication, which hinders judgment and increases the chance of risky sexual behaviors.

We have so many stories about how alcohol and drug addiction affects the whole family. For example, driving when on drugs is extremely unsafe and can cause serious injuries or even death. Same goes for drunk driving, it puts the driver, passengers, and others who share the road at a huge risk. Some people think that one little glass of alcohol won't do any harm; however, even a small amount of alcohol when driving can put you and everyone around you in danger.

What causes addiction? It can be caused by various reasons, such as childhood injuries or traumas, emotional, physical, sexual abuse, depression, anxiety, stress, shame, or guilt. To many people, it is like an escape from reality and their struggles in life.

Has technology affected our quality of life?

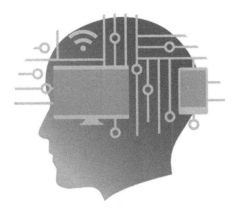

New technologies are being introduced every single day, and with them, new concerns are being introduced as well. According to studies, the average millennial picks up smartphone 150 times a day. This is when we over dependence on technology is known as technology addiction.

Here is a list of common diseases and maladies from excessive use of digital devices:

- Eye strain,
- Tendonitis,
- PlayStation (or Xbox) palmar hidradenitis, a gaming disease with inflammation and red blotches on the palms of your hands after prolonged use of game console controllers,
- Noise-induced hearing loss from prolonged high-volume listening

- Fear of missing out (FOMO) syndrome, characterized by anxiety and stress from fearing that one is missing out on some important experience,
- Nomophobia (no mobile phone phobia), fear and anxiety anytime one is without their cell phone.

Recently the National Institutes of Health started funding the study of Internet and digital device addiction. This is predicted to be a growing area for research as technology becomes more and more central to our everyday lives.

Technology affects attention. Evidence suggests that reliance on the Internet and mobile technology is shortening our attention spans. How many times do we miss important conversations or moments happening around us because we are mesmerized by our electronic device?

Technology affects sleeping. The blue light emitted by screens on cellphones, computers, and televisions restrain the production hormone melatonin that controls your sleep. Reducing melatonin makes it harder to fall and stay asleep. Technology changes the way kids socialize and interact with others, which can have huge impacts on their mental and well-being

Smoking

Smoking is deadly. About one fifth of Americans die, in some way, because of cigarette smoking. The tobacco industry tried to make people believe that smoker can quit whenever they feel like it, that it is solely a matter of personal choice. No matter how you smoke it, tobacco is dangerous to your health. There are unsafe substances in all tobacco products, from acetone and tar to nicotine and carbon monoxide. The substances you inhale affect your entire body. Cigarettes contain about six hundred ingredients, many of which can also be found in cigars and hookahs, according to the American Lung Association, when these ingredients burn, they generate more than seven thousand chemicals. One of the ingredients in tobacco is a mood-altering drug called nicotine. The nicotine in tobacco gets rapidly into your brain and affects the central nervous system and creates addiction and craving. The tobacco industry has designed and modified cigarettes to make them as addictive as possible.

*Smoking effects on the body:*

- Unhealthy teeth
  Yellowing or brownish stains on the teeth increase your risk for infections or inflammation that can lead to tooth and bone loss.
- Respiratory system
  People who smoke are at higher risk for chronic non-reversible lung conditions, such as emphysema, chronic bronchitis, and lung cancer.
- Cardiovascular system
  Nicotine causes blood vessels to tighten, which restricts the flow of blood. Smoking also raises blood pressure, weakens blood vessel walls, increases blood clots, and raises the risk of stroke.
- Digestive system
  Smoking increases the risk of mouth, throat, larynx, and esophagus cancer. Smokers also have higher rates of pancreatic cancer. Furthermore, smoking has an effect on insulin, making it more likely that smokers will develop insulin resistance.
- Sexuality and reproductive system
  Nicotine affects blood flow to the genital areas of both men and women. For men, this can decrease sexual performance. For women, this can result in sexual dissatisfaction by decreasing lubrication and the ability to reach orgasm. Smoking during pregnancy causes problems for both mother and babies.
- Appearance
  Smoking affects your hair, nails, and especially your skin. A substance in tobacco smoke actually changes the structure of skin and increases the risk of skin cancer.

Smoking increases the likelihood of fungal nail infections and has been found to increase hair loss, balding, and graying.

- Heart

    Cigarette smoking is a major cause of stroke. Smoking causes coronary heart disease, the leading causes of death in the United States.

    We have set a no-smoking policy. Get rid of unhealthy habits so you could proudly say, "I am a nonsmoker!"

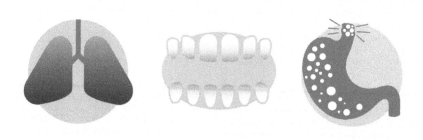

## Summary

The study of disease differences in world populations is unraveling the mystery that most of these modern killer diseases are lifestyle related. They are basically diseases of affluence—too much eating and drinking, too much smoking, addiction to TV and phones, not enough movement and exercise.

Depending on expensive, high-tech medical facilities and equipment for health is not the solution. Studies showing that most diseases are lifestyle related and potentially preventable and reversible are the most important medical discoveries of our time.

My life was affected by World War II, and I was ill since birth. I was looking for a solution. Working in a rehabilitation center, I saw firsthand how people are suffering from illness. I resolved to use my life experience and education to help other people reach their goals, have good relationships, and enjoy life.

Over the last twenty years in the US, I have been educated as a natural health consultant, and I became an energy healer and certified health coach. I believe that nutrition, lifestyle, clean water, and environment and spirituality are the path to good health.

I want to help others understand that each of us is more powerful than any circumstance one could encounter.

# Chapter 2

# Setting Priorities

Sugar is an important source of energy, with glucose being the most important one for the body. However, consuming too much sugar can cause serious health issues. Nowadays so many products contain unhealthy amounts of sugar, which is why overconsumption of sugar is becoming a common and serious issue in our society.

## Sugar

The American Heart Association recommends no more than six teaspoons (25 grams) of sugar per day for women and nine teaspoons (38 grams) for men. Most Americans are consuming way too much sugar—on average, nearly fifty-seven pounds of added sugar per person, every year. Sugar stimulates insulin production, which can cause ability to produce insulin, and this can lead to fat gain and diabetes. The average American consumes 19.5 teaspoons (82 grams) of sugar every day. Children and teens are particularly at risk for fats from added sugar alone. With as many as eleven teaspoons (46.2 grams) of added sugar in one 12 oz. soda, a single serving is close to double most people's daily allowance. According to the Harvard School of Public Health, most sugar in American's diets is added sugar that comes from processed foods. Sweet breakfast cereals, sweets, and sugar-sweetened beverages, such as sodas and fruit juices, contain some of most added sugar of any processed foods; but there is also sugar lurking where you might never expect it to be, foods like ketchup, mustard, salad dressing, and yogurt and granola bars. Using brain-scanning technology, scientists at the US National Institute on Drug Abuse were among the first to show that sugar causes changes in people's brains similar to those in people addicted to drugs such as cocaine, opiates, and alcohol. Too much sugar can increase the over-all risk for heart disease. In fact, sugar actually changes the muscle protein of the heart.

Ten ways sugar harms your health:

1. Sugar causes blood glucose to spike and plummet.
2. Sugar increases the risk of obesity, diabetes, and heart disease
3. Sugar interferes with immune function.
4. A high-sugar diet often results in chromium deficiency.
5. Sugar accelerates aging.
6. Sugar causes tooth decay.
7. Sugar can cause gum disease, which leads to heart disease.
8. Sugar affects behavior and cognition in children.
9. Sugar increases stress.
10. Sugar takes the place of important nutrients.

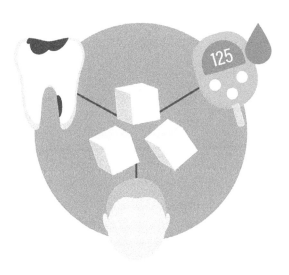

## Meat

Most Americans are meat eaters, relying on beef, chicken, pork, etc., to satisfy most of their protein needs. Meat also supplies nutrients, such as iron and B vitamins, in which many vegetables are deficient. It contains essential fats we need for energy, nerves, and heat insulation. With only six ounces a day of complete protein, we could satisfy most of our protein requirements. However, meat commonly available in our society has so many other drawbacks that you may prefer to gradually eliminate it from your diet. For instance, saturated fat and cholesterol, which are found in high amounts in many meats, increase the hardening of the arteries and heart disease. Consuming meat doubles your chances for colon and rectal cancer while tripling them for breast cancer. The high-protein intake of beef eaters places undue stress on the liver and kidneys, two important organs of detoxification. It may deplete your calcium supply, leading to osteoporosis, and uric acid it contains in the joints, inducing painful gouty arthritis.

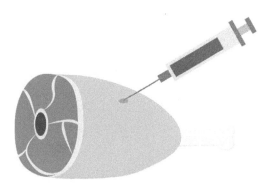

There are hidden poisons in meat and poultry that, when eaten, place undue stress on our digestive systems. These include hormones, antibiotics, tranquilizers, additives, preservatives, and pesticides that are added to the meat in breeding, feeding, and processing the animals. We have blindly assumed, for too long, that so called "healthy"

foods cannot hurt us and that meat is magical. These, quite simply, are myths that have been fabricated and propagated by the meat and dairy industries.

A new study from Harvard School of Public Health (HSPH) in Boston, Massachusetts, found red meat consumption is associated with an increased risk of total cardiovascular and cancer mortality. The results also indicated that substituting other healthy protein sources, such as fish, poultry, nuts, and legumes, was associated with a lower risk of mortality. "This study provides clear evidence that regular consumption of red meat, especially processed meat, contributes substantially to premature death," said Frank Hu, professor of nutrition and epidemiology at HSPH.

Why is meat so bad?

The meat we eat comes from factory farms 99 percent of the time. The meat industry tells consumers that factory farms are modern, efficient, and produce cheap food. What they don't tell you is that factory farms leave consumers with less choices, paying more for dairy, meat, and poultry while the farmer gets paid less, leaving more profit for the middleman. Factory farms increase the risk of pathogens like a e-coli and salmonella that cause food-borne illness in people.

Antibiotics in meat

Factory animals are held in crowded, stressful, and unhealthy living conditions, which is not only inhumane but also requires routine doses of antibiotics. Animals are forced to grow three times faster than natural growth rates.

Due to selective breeding and the use of weight-gaining drugs in feed, animals are forced to grow at an alarming and unhealthy rate. The fact is 80 percent of the antibiotics consumed in the US are used by agriculture. Shockingly, these antibiotics are often used routinely not for treatment of sick animals, but to help them gain weight or prevent disease fostered by their high density, unhealthy, and unsanitary living conditions.

Antibiotics are made to help us heal, but overuse leads to the creation of resistant bacteria, which the CDC considers a top public health threat to the US. Antibiotic resistant bacteria travels from farms through the unsanitary handling of equipment and animals, through airborne dust blowing from the farms, or through water and soil, that has been polluted with contaminated feces. Keeping farm animals healthy and safe is important, but overmedicating is not the answer. The inappropriate use of human antibiotics in agriculture is seen as one of the culprits in the 2 million illnesses and 23,000 deaths caused by drug-resistant bacteria each year in the United States according the Center for Disease Control (CDC).

## Plants

Plants are important sources of products that people use, including food, fibers, medicines. Plants also help provide some of our energy needs. Plants are the only organisms that can convert light energy from the sun into food. They produce all the food that animals, including humans, eat. The animals that give us meat, such as chickens and cows, eat grass, oats, corn, or other plants. Without plants, we wouldn't be able to survive. These days, most plants used for production come from conventional farms. Conventional farms use pesticides for killing insects or weeds.

Pesticides

Pesticides can be very toxic to other living organisms, such as birds, fish, beneficial insects, and even humans. Pesticides can be found in the air, food we eat, and water we drink. They are used almost everywhere these days, which is bad for us and the environment. Herbicides and insecticides, used for plant growing, can cause a long-term chronic illness. Pesticides are bad for the environment as well. For example, they can cause water pollution by traveling through the farmland soil and reaching our drinking water supplies.

Conventional farming allows us to produce much larger quantities of food, on less land and with less manual labor. But it mostly produces commodity crops like corn and soybeans. These crops are used to make processed foods that dominate most people's diet in the US diet. These foods are really bad for our diet and have a great impact on our health. The best solution for us and future generations is to switch from conventional farms to organic gardens.

## Organic Garden

Why organic garden?

In 1945, Albert Howard wrote a book *The Soil and Health.* This book is still relevant today. He says, "Healthy soil gives to healthy plants, which give to healthy people." Most of us think of the soil as tiny pieces of dead rock, but it is much more than that. A tablespoon of healthy soil contains twenty million to two billion beneficial bacteria. Bacteria plays a part in the natural cycling of nutrients and minerals from an unusable form into life-usable forms and back again. We have healthy soil, free from toxic chemicals, which means that the produce is free of toxic chemicals as well. These fruits and vegetables should not have a chemical residue, even if not washed thoroughly.

By planting your own organic garden, you are assuring yourself and your family the best possible fruits and vegetables. Plus, you have the added benefit of exercise, from planting the seeds to carrying in the harvest. Working in your garden will tone your body and work off extra calories. Organic fruits and vegetables also taste better than those you purchase from the supermarket.

Planting your own organic vegetable garden will also save you money. Buying organic produce at farmers markets and health food stores can cost up to 50 percent or more over the regular supermarket. As an added benefit, many people report they have become more spiritual while filling the soil, planting seeds, or pulling weeds in their own garden.

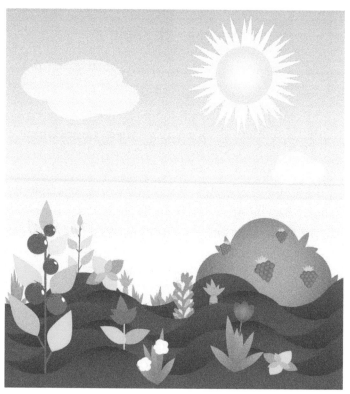

A common quote from those who do gardening:
"It is the time with my higher power."

# Chapter 3

# Detoxification

We are surrounded by toxic substance in the air, water, soil, and food. We now carry in our bodies a modern-day chemical cocktail derived from industrial chemicals, pesticides, food additives, heavy metals, and residues of pharmaceutical, legal, and illegal drugs. Detoxification is the body's natural process of elimination or neutralization of toxins in the liver, the kidneys, urine, and feces.

Dr. Elson Haas, MD, director of the Marin Clinic of Preventive Medicine and Health Education in San Rafael, California says, "The modern diet with excess animal proteins, fats, caffeine, alcohol, and chemicals inhibits the optimum function of our cells and tissues. The cleansing of toxins and waste products will restore optimum function and vitality." Dr. Haas has practiced juice fasting regularly for nearly twenty years and advises his patients to undertake some form of detoxification periodically to clear wastes and dead cells and help the body to function naturally.

How do you start to detoxify?

First you lighten up your toxin load by eliminating alcohol, coffee, cigarettes, refined sugars, and saturated fats. You should also try minimizing the use of chemical-based household cleaners and personal health-care products (cleansers, shampoos, toothpastes) and substitute them with natural alternatives. Next, you need to reduce stress hormones inside your system. Meditation and yoga are really good and healthy ways you can relieve stress. This will help you reset your physical and mental reactions. There are many ways to detoxify your body. Consult your doctor before doing any health treatment, including herbal supplements and natural remedies. Tell your doctor if you have a serious medical condition or are taking any medications.

## Liver Cleanse

By cleansing the liver, you can help one of your most import-ant organs function much better by producing more effective bile. Detoxifying your liver helps it remove toxins and break down fats more successfully. If your doctor has told you that your liver has higher than normal enzyme levels, you drink alcohol regularly, or you sometimes binge drink, your liver is bogged down. Other things that can cause liver problems are high sugar intake, use of chemicals to clean your house, or a diet with too many processed foods. Signs that your liver needs cleansing are dry skin, fluctuating blood sugar readings, and unexplained back pain.

## Liver Cleansing Juice Recipe I

4 medium carrots scrubbed
2 handfuls of baby spinach
1 medium red beet
1 cucumber
1 green apple
1 lemon, skin removed
1 inch of fresh ginger root
A pinch of sea salt

Blend these in a juicer, and you are ready to clean your liver.

# Liver Cleansing Juice Recipe II

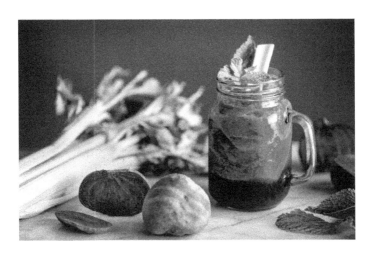

1/2 beet
1/2 cucumber
2 carrots
3 celery stalks
2 stalks of Swiss chard
A handful of parsley

Juice these ingredients and add fresh-squeezed lemon juice to the glass and drink.

# Liver Cleansing Juice Recipe III

1 beet
One handful of washed dandelion greens
1 apple
1 cucumber, peeled
1 lemon peeled

Put all the ingredients in the juicer and enjoy!

Beets are low in calories, high in vitamin C, folate, potassium, and magnesium. Cucumbers are a good source of fiber and are low in calories. Apples and lemons have vitamin C.

## Liver Cleaning with Turmeric

2 apples
3 carrots
3 large celery stalks
3 thumbs of ginger (a thumb
    is about two inches long)
1 lemon, peeled
2 pears
6 thumbs of turmeric

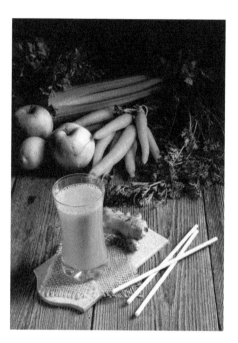

Juice the ingredients and enjoy!

## The One-Day Juice Fast

Juicing is healthy. I rec-ommend the one-day juice fast. Start your day with a cup of warm lemon water. This is 1/2 fresh lemon squeezed in water. After twenty minutes, have a glass of prepared juice. Two hours later, have a cup of herbal tea. For lunch, have another glass of juice. Then two hours later, have a glass of water. Before dinner, have a glass of water and a glass of juice. After a day of fasting, start your seven-day detox diet. In the morning, you drink warm water and juice. The rest of the day you can start eating healthy light food. Each day, for seven days, choose one from the cruciferous family: cabbage, cauliflower, Brussels sprouts, or broccoli. You also need greens such as leafy vegetables and herbs: parsley, kale, Swiss chard, cilantro, beet greens, dandelion greens, and escarole. Then add citrus fruits such as oranges, lemons, and limes (leave out the grapefruit). Other liver healing foods include probiotics such as unsweetened yogurt, sauerkraut, and fermented vegetables, such as kimchi. Spices such as cinnamon, ginger, and nutmeg are not only healthy but delicious too. Ground flaxseeds, olive oil, and flaxseed oil add omega-3 fatty alpha-linolenic acid (ALA), lignans, and fiber, all of which have been shown to have many potential health benefits.

Avoid alcohol and caffeine (coffee, energy drinks, and caffeinated tea.) Stay away from soy, artificial sweeteners, refined carbohydrates, white rice, and anything with white flour, sugars, and especially fried foods and trans fats. Each day, have at least two servings of meat or fish. A serving is about the size of your palm or a deck of cards. Drink eight glasses of filtered water and have two tablespoons of olive or flaxseed oil.

## Natural Colon Cleansing

Colon cleansing is normally used as preparation for medical procedures, such as a colonoscopy. However, some alternative medicine practitioners offer colon cleansing for detoxification. Proponents of colon cleaning believe that toxins from your gastrointestinal tract can cause a variety of health problems, such as arthritis and high blood pressure. They believe that colon cleansing improves health by boosting your energy and enhancing your immune system.

## Colon Cleansing with Powdered or Liquid Supplements

You take some supplements used for colon cleansing through mouth while others you take through the rectum. Either way, the idea is to help the colon to expel its contents. You can find these products in pharmacies or healthy food stores. They include enemas, herbal teas, and magnesium. The instructions are on the packages. You can also do a salt water flush for people experiencing constipation and irregularity. Before eating breakfast, mix two teaspoons of sea salt or Himalayan salt in a glass of warm water. Drink the water quickly on an empty stomach. In a few minutes, you will have an urge to go to the bathroom. Do this in the evening again and make sure to stay home near the bathroom for a while after the cleanse.

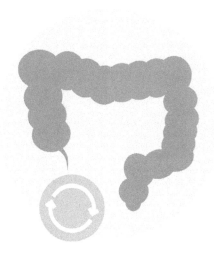

## Dr. Axe's Colon Cleanse

1/2 teaspoon sea salt
1/2 cup 100 percent organic apple juice
2 tablespoons of fresh lemon juice
1 teaspoon ginger juice
1/2 cup warm purified water

Start with a half cup of purified water in a pan, and put it on a low setting. You want it to be warm, not boiling. When it is warm, put it in a glass, and add the sea salt and the rest of the ingredients. Drink it in the morning on an empty stomach. Have the mixture again just before a light lunch and again at midafternoon. Drink additional water that is room temperature.

*This cleanse is safe, but those that are pregnant or have other health issues should check with their doctor before doing any cleanse.*

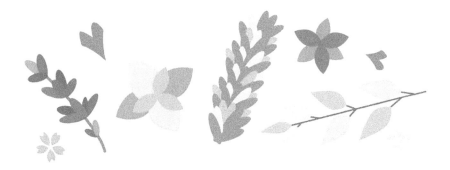

## Detox Your Body with Herbs

Herbs are a natural therapy choice for people concerned with the preservation of the planet. The body has its own process of maintaining a stable environment, and herbs used the right way will not upset the balance of nature. Psyllium is an herb that grows around the world but is mostly found in India. It comes from *Plantago ovata* seeds. The seeds of this plant have been used for thousands of years in traditional medicine. Psyllium soaks up water in the bowels and eases constipation and overall digestive health. It is also a prebiotic and helps probiotics grow in the digestive tract. The bacteria that grows on it will reduce inflammation and aid your immune system. It is used to treat irritable bowel syndrome (IBS) and ulcerative colitis. You can buy psyllium at a health food store. Don't buy the tablet form or powdered form. Get only the whole psyllium husks that you can mix with water, juice, or soy milk. Those over twelve years old can take one tablespoon mixed with eight ounces of liquid. Take this up to three times a day. Avoid alcohol, coffee, or dairy products while cleansing. In addition, make sure to drink five to eight glasses of water a day. If you have Crohn's disease or chronic digestive issues, discuss this with your doctor.

Dandelion (*Taraxacum officinale*)

Dandelion is an herb that has been said to have some detoxification properties. Herbalists have used it for thousands of years.

You can use the flowers, leaves, and even the roots. If you are gathering your own dandelions, make sure not to pick any that are near places where they could be exposed to fertilizer or road chemicals. Dandelion tea is highly efficient when it comes to eliminating toxins from inside the body and has diuretic properties to reduce excess fluids. Dandelion has vitamin K, A, and C. This helps your immune system, blood-clotting ability, and bone health.

There have been some studies of dandelion for use in treating cancer and diabetes. Korean scientists published a study in the *International Journal of Molecular Sciences* that suggested dandelion could regulate blood sugar and insulin levels by helping control fats. You can make a leaf infusion by using 1/2 ounces of dried leaves per cup of boiling water. Steep for ten minutes, then strain. Drink three cups a day. You can make a root decoction by gently boiling two to three teaspoons of powdered root per cup. Boil for fifteen minutes, and then let it cool and strain. Drink three cups per day. People on medications should check with their doctors and pharmacists. This includes people taking water pills and drugs that are changed in the liver. People who have allergies to ragweed or other plants might have a problem with dandelion.

Detox with lemon and cayenne pepper

An excellent healthy alternative detox is lemon water and cayenne pepper drink sweetened with honey. In order to detox, it is recommended that this should be consumed for ten days. It is best to have this drink first thing in the morning. Lemons boost your energy level. Cayenne helps reduce your risk of developing blood clots due to its high concentration of capsaicin. Your best bet to better health is to detox with this drink, and balance this with a healthy diet throughout the day.

*Benefits of detoxing with lemon water and cayenne pepper.* The properties of cayenne pepper and lemon are ideal for detoxing the body when used as a supplement to a healthy lifestyle. A drink of lemon water, honey, and cayenne pepper, consumed daily can provide a wealth of benefits as part of a healthy diet. Much of the health benefits of this natural elixir come from the powerful active ingredients found in both lemon and cayenne pepper. Lemon contains about 8 percent citric acid, which has historically been used as a natural preservative. Not only that, citric acid aids in smooth digestion, helps dissolve kidney stones, and actually helps alkalize the body. Capsaicin in cayenne pepper has been proven to treat anything from headaches to osteoarthritis. Research continues to reveal more wonders of this antioxidant every year. Together lemon and cayenne pepper provide a truly nourishing elixir of health. This is why we should drink lemon and cayenne pepper together.

Benefits include the following:

- *Boosted immunity.*
- *It stimulates the liver.* The combination provides the liver with the right balance of nutrients to detox from harmful substances, such as sugar and alcohol.
- *It aids digestion.* Cayenne pepper stimulates the digestive system and intestines. It soothes gas and takes care of a sour stomach and other digestive problems.
- *It defends against bacteria.* Cayenne and lemon are both powerful allies in the fight against bacteria. This drink can prevent you from becoming sick.
- *It lowers blood pressure.* Cayenne pepper is stimulating the circulatory system to keep your blood pressure low.
- *It helps you fight cravings.* Cayenne helps boost the metabolism, which burns fat while suppressing appetite.
- *It aids the lymphatic system.* Cayenne is a stimulant, so it encourages the cells to work more efficiently.
- *It possibly helps fight cancer.* A 1998 study found that capsaicin has twenty-two anti-cancer properties.
- *It fights viruses.* Cayenne contains compounds that soothe sore throats and reduce congestion. This beverage is ideal for use during cold and flu season.
- *It relieves pain.* The ability of cayenne to dramatically reduce nerve and joint pain has received considerable scientific study.

- *Cayenne prevents blood clots.* Blood clots can be dangerous if left undiagnosed. High concentration of capsaicin in cayenne helps reduce the chance of getting blood clots.
- *It keeps skin healthy.* Cayenne has been used for hundreds of years as a treatment for snake bites, open sores, wounds, bug bites, and many other conditions.

Cayenne pepper weight loss diet plan

You can add 1/2 teaspoon cayenne pepper to many juices or smoothies to lose weight. You can use it in many home-cooked meals. Add 1/2 or 1 teaspoon to salads, soups, yogurt dips, and other food preparations without making its spiciness too overbearing. If you do not want to add it to your food, you can always buy cayenne pepper capsules for weight loss and other health benefits.

When you wake up, you should drink warm water with the juice of lime. At breakfast, have the master cleanse juice (look at the next page for recipe). After the juice, you can eat scrambled eggs plus four almonds, or oatmeal with four almonds. About an hour before lunch, have a cup of green tea. Lunch could be a teaspoon of hummus with a pinch of cayenne pepper and one pita bread.

Evening snack should be around 4:00 p.m. to 4:30 p.m. with a glass of buttermilk, or lentil soup with garlic cayenne pepper and vegetables, or fresh coconut water, or a small bowl of fruit. Dinner should be at 7:00 p.m. with grilled fish with cayenne pepper and cumin powder with vegetables. If you are just getting started with cayenne pepper, go lighter on the amount and work up to using more.

Balance the intake of your detox drink with a healthy diet filled with vegetables and fruits, and you will feel much better!

# The "Master Cleaner Juice" for Weight Loss

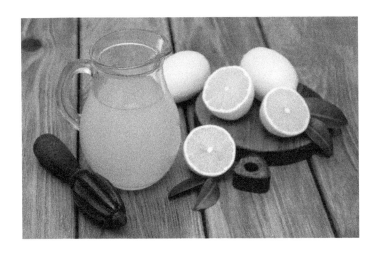

2 tablespoons fresh lemon juice
2 tablespoons grade B maple syrup
A pinch of cayenne pepper
1 cup water

Add all the ingredients to a cup of water. Stir well before drinking.

## Lemon and Cayenne Powder Detox

1 glass of warm water (8–12 ounces)
2 tablespoons of fresh lemon juice
1 tablespoon of raw honey
1 teaspoon of ginger
1 pinch of cayenne pepper

Mix everything and enjoy!

## Cayenne Powder and Cinnamon Detox

A glass of warm water
Juice from 1/2 lemon

2 tablespoons of apple cider vinegar
1 teaspoon cinnamon
1 teaspoon cayenne pepper

This drink can be pretty strong, so make sure you have some water standing by to chase it down. Both drinks help you detox your body naturally.

## Enemas

An enema is an alternative healing method to cleanse the colon. Enemas remove waste and toxins from the colon. Noneliminated waste can build up in the colon and lead to a host of health issues including allergies, bad breath, back pain, and sinus problems. The most common enema is a coffee enema.

## Flush Your Body with Vitamin C

Ascorbic acid is the primary preventative agent of free radical damage. It is needed for proper absorption of many minerals, such as iron and calcium. Research shows that people with a high level of ascorbic acid in their blood live longer than people with low levels. By combining the detoxification of pollutants and toxins with boosting the immune system using vitamin C, a detox flush with ascorbic acid can greatly contribute to longevity. The vitamin C flush involves taking as much vitamin C as your gut can tolerate in order to saturate your body. When you have reached "bowel tolerance" or at the point at which you can no longer absorb vitamin C from your gut, you will experience an evacuation of liquid from your bowels. For this reason, it is important to choose a day to flush when at home and near the bathroom. How does this work? It is important to use ascorbic acid powder or buffered ascorbic acid powder. The buffered version is combined with buffer minerals, such as calcium, magnesium, and zinc.

1. Begin the cleansing first thing in the morning before you eat.
2. Take 1000 mg of vitamin C mixing it into a half glass of water.
3. Repeat this every hour, on the hour, recording each time you take a dose and continue until you need to use the bathroom. The bowel will pass a watery stool. The flush is finished, and you can stop drinking vitamin C.
4. The next time you go to the bathroom, the stools may still be watery but will soon return to normal.

## Detox Diets

Our bodies naturally detoxify every day. This is a normal body process of eliminating toxins from the colon and liver. If your energy level is low, if you have been taking too many medications, your system may not be able to handle all the toxins. It is good to have a detox diet once a season. Here are some examples.

Breakfast protein smoothie with the following:

1. Greens such as spinach, kale, Swiss chard, and dandelion.
2. Liquid such as water, coconut milk, or almond milk.
3. Fruit such as banana, mango, orange, peaches, apples, avocado, blueberries, raspberries, or strawberries.
4. Boosters such as chia seeds, coconut oil, cinnamon, and flax seeds.

There is a variety of detoxification techniques available. Several can be used in combination to improve your well-being and increase your cell awareness. Before you choose to detox, talk to a medical professional to decide what is best for you. Once you complete the cleansing, you should feel fantastic and your face should look rejuvenated. You probably will have lost some weight, and you should feel more energetic.

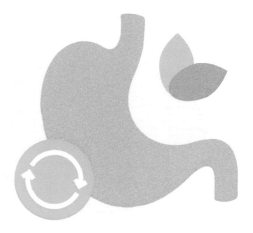

My personal favorite breakfast smoothie.

1 medium banana
1 cup fresh pineapple
3 large handfuls of fresh spinach
1 cup of plain yogurt
6 ounces of water
1 teaspoon of coconut oil.

First blend the greens. Then add fruits and yogurt and blend. After drinking the smoothie, you can have omelet, two eggs, or oatmeal for your breakfast.

# Chapter 4

# Nutrition for Healthy Living

Nutrition is how food affects the health of the body. Food is essential to every living being. It provides vital nutrients for survival and helps energize the functioning of the body.

Food affects your mental alertness and physical well-being. More nutrients mean more fuel to increase your energy level to do more physical tasks. If you pay attention to nutrition facts and strategies, you can take control of your weight. This added attention can bring a longer life span and quality of life.

Nutrient-rich foods such as blueberries, seeds, and avocado can enhance cognitive function. Pumpkin seeds and broccoli have been shown to improve short-term memory due largely to folic acid. Salmon and other fatty fish have long been considered "brain food" because of the omega-3 polyunsaturated fatty acids that improve concentration and retention of facts. Quercetin is a substance found in capers and green tea that stimulates blood flow to the brain. Macronutrients are those nutrients that are required in large amounts to fuel our bodies such as carbohydrates, proteins, and fats. Micronutrients are those nutrients that the body needs in smaller amounts such as vitamins and minerals.

# Carbohydrates

Carbohydrates supply your body with glucose. This is the primary source of fuel for your body and helps you keep up with physical and mental demands and prevent fatigue. Based on a two-thousand-calorie diet, you need 225 grams of carbohydrate according to MayoClinic.com. Carbohydrates include sugar, starch, and fiber.

Carbohydrates are also classed as complex or refined based on how quickly the body absorbs them. Sometimes we need quick release of energy, but we don't need all of them right away. We depend on the complex carbohydrates to keep us going all day. The refined carbohydrates have the outer shells of the grains removed so the fiber and some of the vitamins are removed too. The refining makes it possible to have lighter and prettier foods such as breakfast cereal, pasta, and some breads, at the cost of vital minerals, vitamins, and fiber that improves digestion. The breads that most people eat are 55 percent carbohydrate, since the refined flour is made from 75 percent refined carbohydrates. Most flour cereals are 80 percent refined carbohydrates, and most pastas are 85 percent refined carbohydrate. Candy, jam, jelly, and some pastries are over 90 percent refined carbohydrates. In contrast, fresh fruit is only 15 percent carbohydrate. Dry legumes are 60 percent carbohydrate, and leafy vegetables are a mere 8 percent carbohydrate. The point is, by eating more fruits and vegetables and cutting out refined carbohydrates, we are reducing calories and sugars in our diet. This improves our health. The ideal diet gets most of its calories (85–90) from complex carbohydrates. The rest of the energy comes from fats found in nuts, seeds, and oils. However, most of us do not eat an ideal diet. Many of us overeat, and this causes the body to store this extra energy as fat or liver glycogen. Potato chips are not as good as whole potatoes since they add unnecessary oils. White breads and buns contain little to no fiber plus added sugars that lead to obesity, hypoglycemia, diabetes, and other blood-sugar disorders.

We should improve the quality of our diet by eating more quality carbohydrates. These quality carbohydrates should come from the following:

- Whole grains that have fiber and micronutrients such as potassium, magnesium, and selenium.
- Fiber-rich fruit such as berries, apples, bananas.
- Fiber-rich vegetables including broccoli, leafy greens, and carrots.
- Beans that have fiber, iron, and potassium.

To sum up, eat more whole grains and limit food with added sugars. Stay away from over-processed food and simplify your diet.

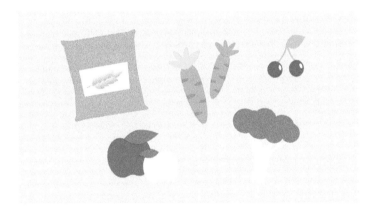

## Protein

Protein is made of large and complex molecules that are critical to the body. Proteins are needed in our cells and are required to support the structure, function, and regulation of the body's tissues and organs. Proteins are made of amino acids that attach to each other in long chains. Proteins are not all the same. They have different combinations of carbon, hydrogen, oxygen, and sulfur. Your body can make eighteen of its own amino acids, but it needs food to make the other eight essential amino acids. If you don't eat the right foods, these essential amino acids can't be created in your body. These include histidine, isoleucine, leucine, lysine, methionine, phenylalanine, threonine, tryptophan and valine. Foods that contain all eight amino acids are called protein. Eggs, meat, fish, grains, legumes, nuts, seeds, vegetables, fruits, and dairy contain complete proteins.

Everyone needs some protein because it is essential to build, repair, and replace muscles, tissues, blood, hair, and nails. Even sedentary adults need protein for these functions, but athletes need it even more. Protein also helps control appetite and weight. Controlled higher protein diets can lead to weight loss and body fat loss while preserving muscle mass. Higher protein diets also are less likely to have weight regain. Protein requirements for adults vary by activity levels. The Mayo Clinic recommends 50–175 grams per day, and the University of Iowa hospitals and clinics recommend 45–70 grams per day. The USDA recommends at least 5–6 ounces of protein in your diet each day. Too little protein causes our bodies to break down tissues and leads to overall deterioration. Some symptoms of protein deficiency are muscle weakness, loss of endurance, fatigue, growth retardation, loss of weight, poor healing, and anemia. Pregnant women must be extra careful to avoid protein deficiency because it will affect the health and growth of the unborn baby.

Too much protein can also be a problem. A study by the United States Department of Agriculture (USDA) found that the average American consumes over 165 percent of the recommended daily amount (RDA) of protein from animal products. Children average 209 percent RDA of protein from animal products. Too much protein can cause people to lose calcium through the urine. This missing calcium is needed by our bones and teeth and leads to "brittle bone disease," also known as osteoporosis. High protein diets provide too much saturated fats, cholesterol, and sodium known to cause heart problems. Your body has to get rid of the extra urea, the nitrogen-containing waste product of protein breakdown. This extra work for your liver and kidneys can be stressful, can make you tired, or cause other problems if you don't drink enough water to flush out the kidneys. This is why so many older people get dangerously dehydrated. Protein deficiency is very uncommon in the United States.

According to statistics, the average American eats 200 pounds of red meat, 50 pounds of chicken and turkey, 10 pounds of fish, 300 eggs, and 250 pounds of dairy products yearly. The animal sources of protein often contain harmful amounts of synthetic hormones, saturated fats, antibiotics, pesticides, nitrates, and other harmful ingredients. We have heard warnings about nasty ingredients in those plump overfed turkeys and the carcinogenic effects of charcoal broiling or frying fatty beef, the residues in milk, and mercury in our fish. It doesn't seem to matter—we still buy these products. Animal foods, when combined with the refined carbohydrates, in our typical American diet have been implicated in increasing our risk of heart disease and arteriosclerosis. Studies show that animal proteins contribute more problems than vegetable sources.

Protein digestion is improved by correct cooking. In my life experience, all grains except buckwheat and legumes must be soaked in cold water before cooking. They should be soaked for 15–20 minutes. The soaking takes out the toxins from harvesting and packing machines. Meat should be soaked in cold water with baking soda to tenderize the meat and remove toxins.

It is important to cook meat slowly and thoroughly because of the microorganisms it contains. Pork can harbor a parasite that can cause trichinosis, if it is not thoroughly cooked. Other meats should be broiled or roasted. It is best to avoid deep fried or overdone protein foods. Milk products are especially sensitive to heat and should not be heated above the boiling point. If you have trouble digesting milk, you might try yogurt, buttermilk, or other cultured milk products.

## Fats

Fats are a necessary nutrient in our bodies. The body needs fats to make cell membranes, synthesize hormone-like compounds, and maintain healthy hair and skin. Our bodies can use fat as fuel and store it in the body for use in the future. However, eating too much fat causes obesity and other health problems, such as fatty liver disease, heart disease, gall bladder issues, sleep apnea, and diabetes.

Bad fats include cholesterol, saturated fat, and trans fat. Many cholesterols and saturated fat come from animal products, such as meat and dairy products. However, our own bodies can create cholesterols, and some people produce more than others. Trans fat is fat that is treated with hydrogen to make foods last longer. Many margarine products are made from trans fat. Commercial bakery products also have trans fat.

Since the 1980s, many experts have recommended our fat intake should be 30 percent or less of our diet. Saturated fat should be no more than 10 percent of the food needed to keep a healthy weight. Eating less animal products will lower our cholesterol intake

You should have your doctor check your cholesterol and follow his advice. Eat low fat meats, fish, and poultry without skin. Lower your consumption of meat and dairy while increasing fruits and vegetables.

## Minerals

Minerals are the building blocks of our bodies. They make bones, teeth tissue, muscle, blood, and nerves. They balance body fluids and spark biological reactions. There's two types: macrominerals or microminerals. We need a large amount of Macro-minerals. These include calcium, magnesium, sodium, potassium, and phosphorus. Conversely we only need trace amounts of micro-minerals. These include boron, chromium, copper, germanium, iodine, iron, sulfur, zinc, and selenium.

Calcium (Ca)

Calcium is the most common mineral in our bodies. The average male has 1,200 grams, and the average female has 1,000 grams in their bodies. Most of that calcium makes up our bones and teeth. The rest helps maintain our heart beat and send nerve signals. Calcium lowers cholesterol levels and helps prevent cardiovascular disease. This mineral also is essential to blood-clotting, and the National Cancer Institute feels it can reduce the risk of colorectal cancer.

Calcium deficiency can lead to the following problems: aching joints, brittle nails, eczema, elevated blood cholesterol, insomnia, muscle cramps, nervousness, numbness in the arms or legs, rheumatoid arthritis, tooth decay, depression, and hyperactivity.

Calcium can be found in milk, dairy, salmon, seafood, and leafy green vegetables. You can get it in almonds, asparagus, blackstrap molasses, brewer's yeast, broccoli, buttermilk, cabbage, cheese, dandelion greens, figs, goat's milk, kelp, oats, prunes, sesame seeds, soybeans, tofu, turnip greens, and yogurt. Even herbs such as alfalfa, burdock root, cayenne, chamomile, chickweed, chicory, flaxseeds, paprika, parsley, peppermint, raspberry leaves, red clover, rose hips, yarrow, and yellow dock contain some calcium.

Every day your body sheds calcium in your urine and feces. This is up to four hundred milligrams a day but can be more if you are under stress. You need to be aware of the interrelationship between calcium, vitamin D, phosphorus, magnesium, and protein. Too much protein can make your body lose calcium. It is best to keep your body less acidic and more alkaline with fruits and vegetables to help keep the calcium you need in your body.

Potassium (K)

Potassium is needed in your body for fluid balance, muscle contraction, and for nerve impulses to work properly. Potassium, in conjunction with other minerals, regulates blood pressure and allows the heart and kidney to function properly. When the level of potassium in blood is too low, you can have muscle cramps, feel weak, or even become paralyzed. This can happen from vomiting, diarrhea, adrenal gland disorder or the use of diuretics. Potassium, in conjunction with sodium, helps form an electrical pump that speeds nutrients into every cell of your body while pushing wastes out. In general, vegetables, fruits, and herbs are far richer sources of potassium than animal foods. Leafy green vegetables are an excellent source. High potassium fruits include bananas, cantaloupes, avocadoes, dates, prunes, dried apricots, and raisins. Whole grains, beans, legumes, nuts, and seeds are also great sources. If your skin and other tissues seem worn out, you may be suffering from a potassium deficiency. Swelling of tissues, constipation, and thinning hair can be signs of potassium deficiency.

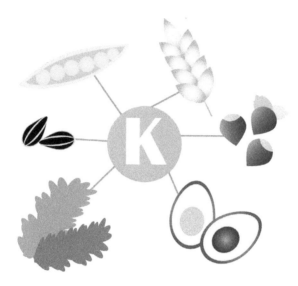

Iron (Fe)

Iron is essential to your body because it is used by blood to transfer oxygen. Hemoglobin transfers the oxygen in the blood, and myoglobin brings oxygen to the muscles. Vitamin C is needed to help the body use oxygen. Iron is available in our diet from animal sources such as beef, veal, pork, lamb, chicken, turkey, fish, shellfish, and liver. It is in plant sources such as greens, tofu, broccoli, sweet peas, kale, Brussels sprouts, cabbage, beets, bean sprouts, and lima beans.

Sodium (Na)

Sodium is a metallic element that occurs in nature only as sodium chloride or salt. Sodium, along with potassium, pumps nutrients into cells and expels waste products. The body needs only a small amount of sodium (less than five hundred milligrams or mg per day) this is less than 1/4 of a teaspoon. Very few people eat less than this amount. Plus, healthy kidneys are great at retaining the sodium that your body needs.

The American Heart Association recommends no more than 2,300 mg a day and moving toward an ideal limit of no more than 1,500 mg per day for most adults. On average, Americans eat more than 3,400 mg of sodium a day. When there is extra sodium in your bloodstream, it pulls water into your blood vessels, increasing the total amount of blood inside them. With more blood in your blood vessels, the blood pressure increases. It is like turning up the water hose for your garden; the pressure inside the hose increases as the amount of water is blasted through it. High blood pressure may overstretch or injure the blood vessel walls and speed the buildup of gunky plaque that can block blood flow. High blood pressure is considered the "silent killer" because the symptoms are not always obvious. Ninety percent of Americans are expected to develop high blood pressure over their lifetimes. Even if you do not have high blood pressure, eating less sodium can help blunt the rise in blood pressure that occurs with age, can also reduce the risk of heart attack, heart failure, stroke, kidney disease, stomach cancer, and even migraines.

More than 70 percent of the sodium we consume comes from packaged, pre-made, and restaurant foods. Some of the sodium in our diet occurs naturally in foods. The remaining sodium in our diet is added by our own cooking. So even if you never touch the salt shaker, you are probably getting too much sodium. One estimate suggested that if Americans lowered their average intake to 1,500 mg/day sodium, it could result in a 25.6 percent overall decrease in blood pressure and an estimated $26.2 billion in health-care savings. Another estimate projected that achieving this goal could reduce cardiovascular disease (CVD) deaths by anywhere from 500,000 to nearly 1.2 million over the next decade.

Selenium (Se)

Selenium is not a mineral that is universally distributed. Some areas of earth have very little. Selenium is a mineral of which we need only trace amounts. The recommended amount of selenium is

70 mcg/day for men and 55 mcg/day for nonpregnant, nonlactating women. Selenium is found in seafood and organ meats primarily, but also in muscle meats, cereals, and other grains and dairy products. The food that is highest in selenium is Brazilian nuts. One nut is 137 percent of the recommended daily intake.

Selenium works at the subcellular level, preventing body fats from going rancid. Rancid body fats are seen externally as age spots or liver spots. This wonderful mineral also inhibits the replication of tumor viruses. Selenium even destroys free radicals and is involved in detoxification of metals.

Dr. Joel Wallach has done research on selenium for about forty years. He states that selenium "may reduce the risk of certain cancers." He has said that selenium deficiency may help prevent oxidative stress that contributes to heart disease, Alzheimer's disease, cancer, premature aging, and stroke. Selenium supplements may help influenza, tuberculosis, HIV, and hepatitis C. However, selenium toxicity is possible and dangerous. It can mean hair loss, dizziness, nausea, vomiting, and in severe cases, heart attack, kidney failure, and death.

Magnesium (Mg)

Magnesium is essential to all living organisms and has electrochemical, catalytic, and structural functions. It activates numerous enzymes and is present in chlorophyll that converts sunlight into chemical energy. The average human body has 20 to 28 grams of total body magnesium. Approximately 60 percent is found in our bones. Twenty-six percent is associated with skeletal muscle, and the balance is distributed between various organs and body fluids. Magnesium is required for the production and transfer of energy for protein synthesis, for contractility of muscle, and excitability of nerves and as a cofactor in a myriad of enzyme processes. Calcium and magnesium have antagonistic roles in normal muscle contraction. Calcium is the stimulator and magnesium is the relaxer. An excessive amount of calcium can induce a magnesium deficiency. Magnesium deficiency diseases can include asthma, anorexia, menstrual migraines, neuromuscular problems, depression, muscular weakness, and calcification of the arteries. Recommended daily intake of magnesium is 350 mg, but 800 mg may be a more realistic figure for maintaining optimal health. Leafy green vegetables are one of the best sources of magnesium. However, you can also get magnesium from nuts, seeds, avocados, whole grains, legumes, organic eggs, honey, and blackstrap molasses.

Zinc (Zn)

Zinc is a mineral that plays a role in growth and sex hormones. It is also involved in the body's utilization of insulin. Zinc helps start many important activities and sparks energy sources. It is an important mineral to keep in a state of balance, keeping your blood at a proper acidity, producing necessary histamines, removing excess toxic metals, and helping kidneys maintain a healthy equilibrium of minerals. Zinc works in the protein production system, blood cells, the circulatory and nervous systems.

You get zinc from eggs, seafood, and organ meats, vegetables including peas, soybeans, mushrooms, whole grains, nuts, seeds, and especially pumpkin. Lack of taste or smell is a sign of zinc deficiency. Acne, psoriasis, and other skin problems can be caused by a lack of zinc. Other signs are brittle hair and bleeding gums. The daily requirement for zinc is 20–25 mg for adults. By including sunflower, sesame, and pumpkin seeds, we can obtain much of our daily requirement for zinc.

Phosphorus (P)

Phosphorus is a mineral found in rocks; however, it gets little or no attention from nutritionists because it is so widely available in all foods. Phosphorus is a major structural mineral for bones and teeth. It is part of most proteins and, as such, may become problematic because elevated phosphorus intake increases calcium requirements when "high protein diets" are consumed. Protein foods like meat, poultry, fish, eggs, dairy products, whole grains, nuts, and seeds supply phosphorus in abundance. Vegetables that contain phosphorus include legumes, celery, cabbage, carrots, cauliflower, string beans, cucumber, chard, and pumpkin. Fruits also contain a healthy supply. Too little phosphorous is responsible for certain anemias. It might also affect your white blood cells and immunity to bacteria and viruses. The recommended daily intake of phosphorus is 800 mg for adults. Pregnant or lactating women need 1,200 mg. If you eat a balanced diet, you should have an adequate amount of phosphorus.

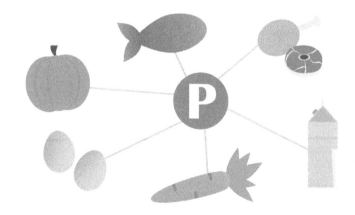

## Vitamins

Vitamins are organic substances that we need to sustain life. The body cannot synthesize vitamins, so they must be obtained in food. The human body can make some of its own vitamin D and K, and the rest come from food or supplements. Vegans may need to supplement their diet with vitamin B12. Vitamins are found only in living things, either plants or animals. Vitamins are essential to the normal functioning of our bodies. They are necessary for growth, vitality, health, general well-being, and for the prevention and cure of many health problems and diseases.

There are thirteen vitamins needed by the human body. These include vitamins A, C, D, E, K, and B vitamins including B1 (thiamine), B2 (riboflavin), B3 (niacin), B4 (adenine), B5 (pantothenic acid), B6 (pyridoxine), B7 (biotin), B8 (inositol), B9 (folic acid),

B10 (para-amino benzoic acid or PABA), B11 (folic acid) and B12 (cobalamin).

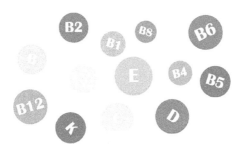

VITAMINS

Water-soluble vitamins

Vitamin B and C are water-soluble and are readily excreted from the body. In fact, urinary output can be a strong predictor of vitamin consumption. Because they are not able to be stored in the body, a consistent daily intake is important. These vitamins can be lost by overcooking. The B vitamins affect the building of enzymes.

Fat-soluble vitamins

Fat-soluble vitamins are absorbed through the intestinal tract with the help of lipids. Because they are more likely to accumulate in the body, they are more likely to lead to hypervitaminosis than are water-soluble vitamins. Fat-soluble vitamins are stored in the liver or fat tissue until needed. The fat-soluble vitamins are A, D, E, and vitamin K.

Vitamin A (retinol)

Vitamin A is important for vision, reproductive function, and normal cell reproduction. It is also important to bone growth and for keeping the mouth, nose, throat, and lungs moist. Vitamin A is an antioxidant that may play a role in the prevention of certain cancers.

Beta-carotene, a precursor to Vitamin A, helps to fight disease-causing free radicals. It is found in milk products, organ meats, and fish oils. Beta-carotene is found in colorful vegetables and fruits including carrots, pumpkin, broccoli, spinach, and sweet potatoes. The color orange or dark green is often associated with beta-carotene.

Lack of vitamin A can cause night blindness and keratomalacia, an eye condition in which the cornea (color part of the eye) becomes dry, cloudy, and soft.

Vitamin B1 (thiamin)

Vitamin B1 or thiamin processes carbohydrates into energy and is necessary for cell function. It has a role in heart function and glucose metabolism.

Thiamin is found in cereal grains, sunflower seeds, brown rice, whole-grain rye, asparagus, kale, cauliflower, potatoes, oranges, liver, and eggs. Overcooking can destroy thiamin. Those that drink a lot of coffee or tea need to be concerned because the tannins in those drinks destroy thiamin. Vitamin B1 supplements have been proven to help people with AIDs, canker sores, cataracts, glaucoma, peripheral neuritis, cervical cancer, diabetic pain, heart disease, kidney disease, and stress. Some athletes use thiamin to boost their performance. Since this is a natural substance, it is legal. Deficiencies of thiamin include beriberi and Wernicke-Korsakoff syndrome (a disease affecting people with chronic alcoholism). Women who have severe morning sickness may also have a need to take a thiamin supplement.

Vitamin B2 (riboflavin)

Riboflavin helps with growth and overall health. It helps break down carbohydrates, proteins, and fats with other B vitamins and allows oxygen to be used by the body. It helps the body absorb oxygen. Vitamin B2 protects glutathione (an antioxidant in the eye). Riboflavin is needed to change vitamin B6 and B9 into other substances the body can use. Riboflavin also processes iron to make red blood cells.

Good sources of riboflavin include beef liver, oats, clams, apples, mushrooms, chard, cottage cheese, milk, yogurt, meat, eggs, fish, bananas, and green beans.

Deficiencies can cause anemia, lip sores, inflammation of the skin, and swelling of the soft tissue of the mouth. The tongue turns a magenta color. This is called ariboflavinosis. It is more common in the places of the world, such as Asia and the West Indies that depend on corn, potatoes, or rice as their main food since these plants don't have riboflavin.

Vitamin B3 (niacin)

Niacin helps control cholesterol, processes alcohol, converts carbohydrates to energy, and maintains healthy skin. Sources of niacin include liver, heart, kidney, chicken, beef, tuna, salmon, milk, eggs, avocados, dates, tomatoes, leafy vegetables, broccoli, carrots, sweet potatoes, potatoes, asparagus, nuts, whole grains, legumes, mushrooms, and brewer's yeast. Breads and cereals are often enriched with niacin.

Deficiency of niacin is a serious condition called pellagra. This disease has a scaly rash on the skin, mouth sores, vomiting, diarrhea, headache, depression, memory loss, and apathy. If untreated, it can be fatal.

Vitamin B4 (adenine)

Adenine is one of the lesser vitamins that are left out of supplements. It speeds up the process by which energy is made in our body and is a component of DNA and RNA. It is found in cereals and bread, honey, bee pollen, as well as eating herbs, vegetables, and fruit.

Vitamin B5 (pantothenic acid)

B5 or pantothenic acid aids in converting fats to energy and synthesizing cholesterol. It is found in milk, eggs, poultry, avocado, mushrooms, legumes, whole grains, organ meats, and cruciferous vegetables, such as cabbage and kale.

Vitamin B6 (pyridoxine)

Pyridoxine is important in the production of hormones such as serotonin, dopamine, and melatonin. It also helps process amino acids. The Mayo Clinic says it is important for brain development and keeping the nervous system functioning properly. It also works with the immune system of the body.

People that have kidney disease, some genetic disease, or epilepsy may need supplements for pyridoxine. A Mayo Clinic report states that some studies show that B6 works with B9 and B12 to control high levels of homocysteine in the blood and that a supplement may help prevent stroke, but more research is needed. There are some studies looking in to the use of B6 for morning sickness and premenstrual symptoms (PMS) but not enough to recommend supplements. Pyridoxine is found in nuts, meat, poultry, bananas, avocados, legumes, and whole grains. Milling and processing of whole grains does remove a big amount of the B6.

Vitamin B7 (Biotin)

Biotin is needed to metabolize fats and turn it into glucose for energy. It also contributes to healthy hair, skin, and nails. However, it cannot be absorbed topically into the hair and skin. Some have called it vitamin H because hair and skin both start with H in German and many chemists have studied German. Studies are taking place to connect biotin with the secretion of insulin and help with diabetes. A deficiency in biotin can lead to hair loss, a scaly rash on the face and genitals, cracks around the corners of the mouth, a tongue that is magenta in color, dry eyes, and the loss of appetite. It also might include depression, insomnia, tiredness, hallucinations, and susceptibility to infections. Patients with Crohn's disease may need to take supplements of biotin because they can't properly absorb it from food.

Biotin is found in peanuts, liver, yeast, bread, cheddar cheese, salmon, pork, sardines, raspberries, avocados, mushrooms, egg yolks, and cauliflower. Egg whites interfere with the absorption of biotin.

Vitamin B8 (inositol)

Inositol is another one of the lesser vitamins not put in supplements. It helps process fat in our liver. It supplies serotonin to the nerves in the brain. It is being studied for treatment of depression, bipolar disorder, and panic disorder. Sources of B8 are whole grains, nuts, and legumes.

Vitamin B9 (folic acid)

Folic acid or folate is a substance needed to help support the adrenal system and a proper brain and nervous system. Pregnant women need it to have healthy babies. Deficiencies can cause depression, low birth weight, pregnancy loss, memory loss, and cervical dysplasia. Alcoholics may need folic acid supplements because alcohol interferes with absorption.

You can get folic acid in your diet from green vegetables and beans, bananas, melons, lemons, yeast, and mushrooms. There are also fortified products such as orange juice, baked goods, and cereals.

Vitamin B10 (para-aminobenzoic acid)

Vitamin B10 or PABA (para-aminobenzoic acid) is more known as a sunscreen ingredient than something we need to add to our diet. It guards our skin from free radicals in harmful chemicals. PABA is contained in leafy vegetables, whole grains, molasses, wheat germ, mushrooms, and eggs. It aids with protein metabolism and the making of red blood cells. It can also be an anti-aging agent to reduce wrinkles and spots on the skin. Since it helps the growth of microorganisms in our body, it can help with irritable bowel syndrome (IBS) and other stomach issues.

Vitamin B11 (salicylic acid)

Salicylic acid works with B12 to form DNA and RNA. It is essential to a growing baby's brain and spinal cord. It is used in skin creams to control acne and skin problems such as psoriasis. It is one of the vitamins not used in supplements. It is commonly found in egg yolk, meat, poultry, potatoes, and leafy green vegetables.

Vitamin B12 (cobalamin)

Cobalamins or B12 are needed for metabolism in the human body. They help with red blood cells and DNA synthesis.

Pernicious anemia is an autoimmune disease that can cause B12 deficiency. If it is not treated, permanent nerve damage can occur. Vitamin B12, folate, and vitamin B6 are involved in homocysteine metabolism. Without enough of these three vitamins, damage can cause vascular disease or diabetes.

Researchers are looking for connections to Alzheimer's disease and dementia. Metformin, a drug to treat diabetes, can reduce the absorption of vitamin B12.

Vitamin B12 is naturally found in animal products, including fish, meat, poultry, eggs, milk, and dairy products. Clams are one of the highest sources, followed by liver. Vitamin B12 is generally not present in plant foods, but fortified breakfast cereals are a readily available source of vitamin B12 with high bioavailability for vegetarians. Some nutritional yeast products also contain vitamin B12.

Vitamin C (L-ascorbic acid)

Vitamin C is important in wound healing and acts as an antioxidant. It also helps the body absorb iron and protein. Research is being conducted to see if vitamin C helps with delaying the development of cancers and cardiovascular disease. Lack of vitamin C causes scurvy. Most people think of oranges and orange juice when they think of vitamin C. It is found in other citrus fruits, as well as potatoes, greens, broccoli, red pepper, spinach, cabbage, tomatoes, cauliflower, strawberries, and Brussels sprouts.

Vitamin D (D2 [ergocalciferol] and D3 [cholecalciferol])

Vitamin D is called the sunshine vitamin because we can manufacture it in our bodies if we are exposed to sunlight. It helps the body absorb calcium and is added to milk products. It can also be found in cereal and fish (cod liver oil.) Vitamin D also helps with cell growth, neuromuscular and immune function, and reduction of inflammation.

Lack of vitamin D can cause rickets in children and poor bone health or osteomalacia in adults. Those with inflammatory bowel disease, liver disease, cystic fibrosis, celiac disease, and Crohn's disease need supplements because their bowels do not properly absorb the vitamin. Obese people or those that had gastric bypass surgery may also need supplements.

It is possible to have too much vitamin D in your system. This can cause kidney stones, anorexia, weight loss, polyuria, and heart arrhythmias. Drugs such as prednisone or drugs used for weight loss or epileptic seizures affect how the body absorbs vitamin D.

Vitamin E

Vitamin E helps our skin, brain, blood, vision, and reproduction. It is also a defense against free radicals in our body that cause heart disease, cancer, and other diseases.

Vitamin E is found in avocado, seeds, nuts, papaya, mango, wheat germ, oils, margarine, spinach, broccoli, asparagus, and turnip greens.

Vitamin E deficiency can cause neuropathy. It also causes pre-eclampsia in pregnant women. However, too much vitamin E can increase the risk of prostate cancer and cause insulin resistance.

Vitamin K (K1 [phytonadione], K2 [menaquinone])

Vitamin K is what makes our blood clot. It is also used to treat conditions where we have bleeding such as spider veins, bruises, and scars. Some medications cause bleeding, such as salicylates, sulfonamides, and some antibiotics; so vitamin K is prescribed. It helps relieve itching from biliary cirrhosis. Along with vitamin D3, it helps some people with psoriasis.

Vitamin K is found in cabbage, cereals, cauliflower, fish, liver, beef, eggs, spinach, kale collards, turnip greens, broccoli, Brussels sprouts, and cilantro.

# Water

The Bible speaks of God's Word about water.

> To make her holy, cleansing her by the washing with water, through the word. (Ephesians 5:26, KJV)

> For as the rain and the snow come down from heaven, And do not return there without watering the earth And making it bear and sprout, And furnishing seed to the sower and bread to the eater; So will My word be which goes forth

from My mouth; It will not return to Me empty,
Without accomplishing what I desire, And with-
out succeeding in the matter for which I sent it.
(Isaiah 55:10–11, NASB)

The Bible speaks of purification and cleansing power of water:

I will sprinkle clean water on you and you will be
clean. I will cleanse you from all your impurities
and from all your idols. (Ezekiel 36:25, KJV)

The average human body is 70 percent water. We start out life being 99 percent water, as fetuses. When born, we are 90 percent water; and by the time we reach adulthood, we are down to 70 percent. In other words, throughout our lives, we exist mostly as water. From a physical perspective, humans are water.

Since humans are 70 percent water, we have to purify the water in the United States. Water in a river remains pure because it is moving. When water is trapped, it dies. Water must be constantly circulated. The water or blood in the bodies of the sick is usually stagnant. Dr. Masaru Emoto discovered that crystals formed in frozen water reveal changes when specific concentrated thoughts are directed toward them. He found that water from clear springs and water that had been exposed to loving words showed brilliant, complex, and colorful snowflake patterns. Polluted water or water exposed to negative thoughts form incomplete asymmetrical patterns with dull colors. Research creates a new awareness of how we can positively impact our personal health.

Water makes up more than two thirds of the human body weight. Without water, we would die in a few days. The human brain is made up of 95 percent water. Blood is 83 percent water, and lungs are 90 percent. A mere 3 percent drop in our body's water supply can trigger signs of dehydration: fuzzy short-term memory, trouble performing basic math, and difficulty focusing on smaller print, such as text on the computer screen. Mild dehydration is also one of the most common causes of daytime fatigue. An estimated seventy-five percent of Americans have mild, chronic dehydration.

Water serves as a lubricant.

Water serves as a lubricant in digestion and almost all other body processes. The water in our saliva helps facilitate chewing and swallowing, ensuring that our food will easily slide down the esophagus. Water also lubricates our joints and cartilages and allows them to move more fluidly. When dehydrated, our body rations water away from the joins. Less lubrication equals greatest friction and that can cause joint, knee, and back pain, potentially leading to injuries and arthritis. Even our eyeballs need plenty of lubrication to work well and remain healthy. Water removes harmful toxins and waste from the body through urination and perspiration.

Water transports valuable nutrients to the body.

Blood is about 92 percent water and carries nutrients and oxygen throughout the body. Nutrients from the food we eat are broken down in the digestive system where they become water soluble, which means they are dissolved in water. Drinking eight glasses of water daily can decrease the risk of colon cancer by 45 percent, bladder cancer by 50 percent, and can potentially even reduce the risk of breast cancer.

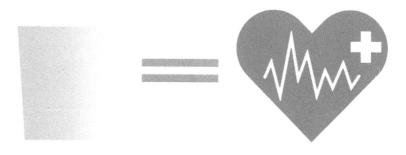

# Chapter 5

# Options for Growing and Finding Healthy Foods

The human body is a complex organism with the ability to heal itself, if you listen to it and respond with proper nourishment and care.

## How to Know What Food We Need

Individual nutrients differ in form and function and in the amount needed by the body. However, they are all vital to our needs. If we do not give ourselves the proper nutrients, we can impair the body's normal functions and cause ourselves great harm. Even if we show no signs of illness, we are not necessarily healthy.

Good nutrition is the foundation of good health. Everyone needs the four basic nutrients—water, carbohydrates, proteins, and fats—as well as vitamins, minerals, and micronutrients. It is important to be able to choose the proper foods and to better understand what foods and where to buy your food. What seems like the smallest choices are truly the keys to changing our lives.

People are hypnotized by theories. Nutrition information is taken from the media: newspapers, books, the web, or magazines. When a specific diet does not work for one person, it brings on a sense of failure. I learned from my studies that there is no perfect diet that works for everyone. I encourage you to explore what works best for you and to trust your body. You are not going to fail at a diet that you create for your unique self. We are a society that wants a pill for every ill. By slowing down and allowing yourself the rest you need, your body has the opportunity to heal on a deeper level.

## How Can Someone Determine the Optimal Diet for Themselves

Some people focus on being very careful about eating while others have a more relaxed attitude toward food. Some people are healthy eating animal products while others thrive on a vegetarian or vegan diet. Human beings know that what they eat changes everything. Over time, people experimented, made mistakes, and slowly have begun to realize that diets do not really work. You can't tell people what kind of relationship to be in or what kind of movies and music they are going to enjoy. Why is it acceptable to tell people what kind of food they should be eating? Food must be about the individual and not about the theory. One person's food is another person's poison.

## What Factors Determine What We Need to Eat.

1. *One factor is gender.* What works for women may or may not work for men. People can become ill by having certain dietary choices forced or pressured on to them.
2. *Another factor is age.* Infants need different foods than young adults or the elderly. Consider the fuel you require to help determine your future.
3. *Culture has an effect too.* Everyone has a genetic predisposition to eat the foods from the country where their ancestors grew up.

## Cravings

Your age, culture, and gender also link to cravings. Understand how to deconstruct cravings by experimenting with similar foods or take small amounts into your diet. No matter what lifestyle you have, no matter what disease you may have, these recommendations will help everyone get well.

1.  Less meat, milk, sugar, and "chemicalized" artificial junk food
2.  Less coffee and alcohol
3.  More fruits, vegetables, and whole foods
4.  Appropriate protein
5.  Enough drinking water
6.  Adequate rest

## Avoid GMOs

Most sources of GMO health information on the web show that GMOs are unhealthy. Human studies show how genetically modified (GM) food can leave material inside of us, possibly causing long-term problems. Genes inserted into GM soy, for example, can transfer inside of bacteria living inside of us. GMO crops require huge amounts of chemicals that are harmful to soil and water by the Department of Agriculture (USDA). In 2008, GMO crops used 26 percent more pesticides per acre than non-GMOs. Research has shown that laboratory mammals fed GMOs suffer adverse effects that include damage to kidneys, liver, adrenal glands, spleen, and heart. Additionally, their immune systems were compromised, and in some, brain size was reduced.

GMOs lead to corporate control over seeds and foods.

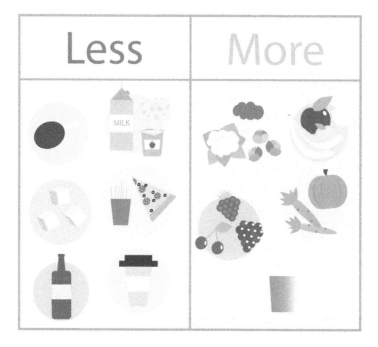

Today only one company controls about 95 percent of GM seeds. This limits access to seeds, which are the center of food and life.

The American Public Health Association and American Nurses Association are among the many medical groups that condemn the use of GM bovine growth hormone because milk from treated cows has more of the hormone IGF-1 (insulin-like growth factor 1) which is linked to cancer.

How can we avoid GMOs that are in 80 percent of all processed food? The only way to stay away from GMOs is to buy certified organic food.

## Reasons to Buy Local Foods

Locally grown food tastes better and looks better. The crops are picked at their peak and farmstead products like cheese are hand-crafted for best flavor. Livestock products are processed in nearby facilities, and typically the farmer has a direct relationship with processors, unlike animals processed in large industrial facilities. Local food is better for you. The shorter the time between the farm and your table, the less likely it is that the nutrients will be lost from fresh food. Food imported from far away is older and has traveled on trucks or planes and sat in warehouses before it gets to you. Local food is safe. There is a unique kind of assurance that comes from looking a farmer in the eye at a farmer's market or driving by the fields where your food comes from. Local farmers take their responsibility to the consumer seriously.

Local food preserves genetic diversity. In the modern agricultural system, plant varieties are chosen for their ability to ripen uniformly, survive packing, and last a long time on the shelf; so there is limited genetic diversity in large-scale production. Smaller local farms, in contrast, often grow many different varieties of crops to provide a long harvest season, an array of colors, and the best flavors.

Fresher food tastes better. Food is picked and eaten at the peak of freshness. It retains more nutrients and tastes better. By choosing food produced locally, you are supporting your community, and you help keep local producers in business. It is good advice to use community-supported agriculture (CSAs) programs. This allows people to purchase seasonal produce directly from local farmers. Usually a CSA-participating farm will offer a certain number of "shares" to the public. The farm will commit to growing food for participating members. Community members, in turn, agree to support the farm through financial contributions, which are typically paid up front. Membership dues help to pay for seeds, plants, greenhouses, utilities, equipment, and labor. Members receive a weekly or biweekly share of the farm's harvest. The community members become shareholders in the farm, and the farm has a steady supply of revenues it can count on. Some CSAs offer home delivery options. Some distribute shares at farmer's markets, and others require members to pick up their shares directly at the arm. At some farms, members get to choose what kinds of products they want in their share each week while other farms let the week's harvest dictate what will be included.

More and more people want to know where food comes from and the farming practices of the farmers that grow and produce it. And this is important for many reasons:

-   It helps you develop a connection with food.
-   You become more aware of your food.
-   You become more aware of what you are putting in your body.
-   You vote every time you shop, and with knowledge comes the ability to support foods and growers you believe in.

## Reading Food Labels

We all have the right to know what is in our food, how it is produced, and where it is from. Food companies are often not required to give us the information we want to know. The current rules in food labeling leave a lot of room for vague claims that make it difficult to differentiate between food produced by sustainable farmers using humane practices and corporate agribusiness green-washing their products. Reading labels can help you make food choices. The labels on processed and packaged foods and drinks in cans, boxes, and jars have a lot of nutrition and food safety information.

Nutrition facts

The nutrients that are listed first are the ones Americans generally eat in adequate amounts. They are identified in yellow color.

The serving size:

The first place to start when you look at the nutrition facts label is the serving size and the number of servings in the package. The size of the serving on the food package influences the number of calories and the nutrient amount listed on the top part of the label. Pay attention to the serving size, especially how many servings there are in the food package. Think, *How many servings am I consuming (1/2 serving, 1 serving, or more)?* Calories provide a measure of how much energy you get from a serving of this food. Most Americans consume more calories than they need without meeting recommended intakes for a number of nutrients. The calorie section of the label can help you manage your weight.

There is a general guide to calories:

- Forty calories is low.
- One hundred calories is moderate.
- Four hundred calories or more is high.

Look at the calories on the label and compare them with the nutrients they offer. Eat less sugar. Food with added sugars may provide calories, but few essential nutrients. Look for foods and beverages low in added sugars. Read the ingredient list and make added sugars are not one of the first few ingredients.

Know your fats. Look for foods low in saturated fats, trans fats, and cholesterol. This will help reduce the risk of heart disease. Most of the fats you eat should be polyunsaturated and monounsaturated fats, such as those in fish, nuts, and vegetable oils. Fat should be in the range of 30 percent to 35 percent of the calories you eat.

How food labels are useful

These labels tell you something meaningful about your food and where it came from, though they may not mean what you think. For example, "certified organic" is a specific government requirement in the US Department of Agriculture organic seal. For a product to be certified organic, it is required to meet specific standards:

- Organic crops can't be grown with synthetic fertilizers or synthetic pesticides.
- Organic crops can't be genetically engineered or irradiated.
- Animals must have access to the outdoors.
- Animals can't be cloned.

However, the USDA organic seal does not show all the information about where the food was made or grown. There are labels such as "grass fed" that means the animals' primary source of food comes from grass, not from grains, such as corn or soy beans. There are no uniform government standards for this label. This does not tell you if antibiotics or hormones were used on the animal.

Missing GMO labels

Many of the processed foods available in our grocery stores include genetically altered ingredients. GMOs have been altered at the genetic level by adding genetic material from different species that could not happen through traditional breeding.

Reduce sodium (salt) and increase potassium

Research shows that eating less than 2,300 milligrams of sodium (about one teaspoon of salt) per day may reduce the risk of high blood pressure. If you are an older adult, try to eat no more than 1,500 milligrams of sodium each day and take at least 4,700 milligrams of potassium. You can get potassium from green vegetables, sweet potatoes, plain yogurt, bananas, and beans. Most sodium comes from processed foods, not from the saltshaker. Read the label and choose foods lower in sodium and higher in potassium.

Look for organic food

Organic food has become very popular. Organic food can't be produced with synthetic ingredients. It must adhere to the standards of the United States Department of Agriculture (USDA) that crops are grown without synthetic pesticides or fertilizer. Some synthetic fertilizer has phosphogypsum that has some naturally occurring radioactive material. Animals grown on organic farms eat organically grown feed and are raised without pesticides.

Organic foods may have a higher nutritional value than conventional food. And those foods that have pesticides, even low levels, can be significantly more toxic for fetuses and children. Staying with eating only organic food keeps GMOs out of your diet and GMOs are used in conjunction with harmful chemicals such as Roundup or Agent Orange.

Shopping organic is taking a stance against the large chemical-producing corporations that have polluted the world's food and fields.

Weeds can be controlled naturally by using methods such as crop rotation, hand weeding, and mulching. We do not need to give our livestock hormones. Pests can be prevented with natural methods such as birds, insects, and traps or using natural pesticides. Organic meat, dairy, and eggs are all given hormone and GMO-free food. Disease is prevented with natural methods, such as a healthy diet, fresh air. Livestock must have access to the outdoors. Organic foods are often more nutrient rich. Organic foods get their nutrients straight from healthy and rich organic soil. In the healthy soil, we do not need to add synthetic fertilizers. Organic foods are more flavorful. The meat of a stressed animal is not as tasty and tender as the meat of a relaxed animal. Organic farming maintains not only your health, but also affects the health of the earth. Organic food is the best gift you can give yourself and your family.

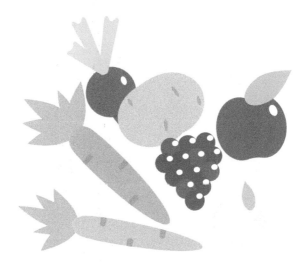

# Cook at Home

Since I was ten years old, I had to prepare meals for my family. After World War II, my country, Lithuania, we did not have many choices for food. I enjoyed cooking. I dreamed that someday I would find an opportunity for everyone to have enough food. I kept the tradition of cooking for my family. I have always cooked for my children, and while they lived with me, they always had home-cooked meals. My family chooses not to eat out very often because they do not know what is in the food.

Even if you are not a great cook, you can cook at home and practice your way to perfection. Cooking at home will help you save money. Restaurants charge a lot for their food. For the cost of eating one meal out, I can feed my family for three days! And leftovers can help you save even more.

Save time

Cooking at home saves precious time. A simple recipe such as rice and stewed chicken can be prepared in 30 minutes. Everyone will be happy to have their food at an appropriate time. No wasted time traveling to the restaurant and no waiting in line for a table is required. Why not cook at home and enjoy the comfort of your own house!

Healthier ingredients

When we prepare our own food, we know exactly what ingredients are in the food and how much of each ingredient is in the food. Commercially prepared foods are high in fat, salt, and sugar. Cooking at home allows you to avoid food allergens and sensitivities. Because you are in control in your own kitchen, you can reduce the risk of an allergic reaction. You can avoid the ingredients in the food you prepare.

Portion control

Many restaurants give very large portions to make you come back again and again. Fast-food places want to supersize your meal to make more money. At home, you control the size of the portions and are less likely to supersize your waist.

Brings the family together

Studies show that when a family eats together, the family members are healthier and happier. Children learn healthy eating habits and learn to talk to others at the table. Home-cooked meals are fresher, taste better, look better, and fill your stomach happily. Let's use our kitchens to prepare meals for our family and enjoy the smells of tasty food in our house!

## Home Gardening

Home gardening gives so many benefits for us by providing vegetables and fruit for your table and beautiful flowers to decorate your home. Gardening offers a variety of health benefits. The National Institute of Health website found that exposure to sunlight helped adults achieve adequate serum vitamin D. Gardening helps to keep our minds sharp in multiple ways. It slows aging by keeping us physically fit doing garden chores and keeping our minds active. Gardening is an activity that almost anyone can do to some degree. A 2006 study found that gardening can lower the risk of dementia. It fights stress better than other hobbies. Gardening gives fresh-picked fruit and vegetables. You know exactly when it is picked and how fresh it is. At the grocery store, you have no idea when it was picked. You have to waste gasoline and time to drive to the store. You can grow your own organic vegetables. You can make your yard inviting. Vegetables and fruit can add life, color, and beauty to your backyard. The smell of basil, mint, and other plants will fill the air. The beauty of ripe tomatoes and cucumbers will be a warm invitation in your kitchen. Plants that sprout beautiful flowers encourage the pollination. Beans, peas, and fruit can make a splash in your yard. Working in the garden will decrease stress and reduce high blood pressure. It can even lower your chance of heart disease.

*Let's start gardening! Everyone can do it!*

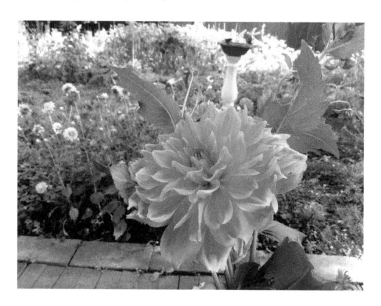

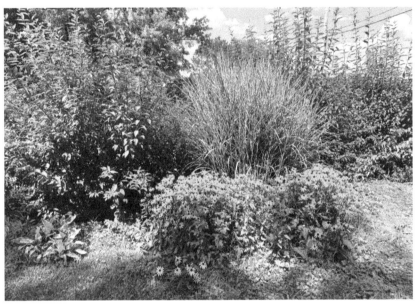

My own garden:

*Flowers from your own garden smell sweeter and the fruits, vegetables, and herbs taste much better when you tend to them with your own hands!*

## Chapter 6

# Healthy Recipes for Cooking at Home

*Creating healthy and delicious foods is easier than one may think. You will soon be making meals that are very nutritious and tasty. Cooking for yourself and loved ones becomes easier over time, and many find great joy in their cooking and learning.*

*Many meals begin with a salad. We will do the same. Salads help one digest their food. They are popular all over the world. Here are some salad recipes that taste great and are very good for you!*

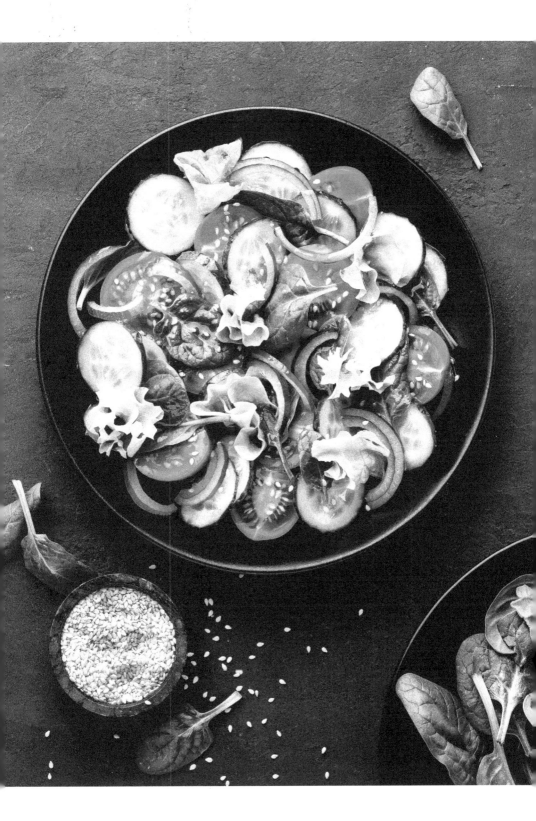

# Sweet Potato Avocado Salad

2 sweet potatoes baked with coconut or olive oil
1/4 cup of quinoa cooked
1 ripe avocado diced
1/3 cup of chickpeas
1 handful of fresh spinach

After sweet potatoes and quinoa are cooked, mix all the ingredients together.

# Kale and Cranberry Salad

2 handfuls of kale chopped
1 carrot grated
1/2 teaspoon of ground black pepper
Juice from half lemon
1/4 cup of dried cranberries
1 tablespoon of chia seeds
1/4 cup of pumpkin seeds
2–3 tablespoons of olive oil

Mix everything and enjoy!

# Beet Salad

2 medium red beets
1 medium Chioggia beet
1 orange
A bag of pre-washed arugula
1/2 red onion (sliced)
1/2 cup of dry and roasted hazelnuts (chopped)
1/2 cup crumbled feta cheese
2 tablespoon white raspberry balsamic vinegar
1 tablespoon brown sugar
Salt and pepper to taste

Preheat oven to 400 degrees Fahrenheit. Wash and cut the ends of the beets (removing greens and stems). Wrap whole beets in foil, bake 45 minutes, and allow to cool. Peel orange and slice into segments. Slice red onion. Place orange segments and red onion in bowl. Add balsamic vinegar. Combine and chill in refrigerator for 10 minutes. Meanwhile, remove the cooled beats from the foil, then peel and slice them.

In a saucepan, add sliced beets, sugar, vinegar. Simmer and stir until sugar is dissolved Place warm beets in a bowl and allow to cool. Coarse chop hazelnuts.

Place arugula, arrange beets and red onions atop arugula. Add hazelnuts and feta cheese. Drizzle remaining raspberry vinegar over salad.

## Butternut Squash Orzo Salad

2 1/2 cups diced butternut squash
1 1/2 tablespoon olive oil
1 cup orzo pasta (uncooked)
2 cups fresh spinach diced
1/2 cup dried cranberries
2 ounces gorgonzola cheese (crumbled)
1/4 cup real maple syrup
1/4 teaspoon salt
1 teaspoon Dijon mustard
1/4 teaspoon pepper
1/4 cup olive oil

**Directions**

Preheat oven to 425 degrees Fahrenheit. Mix diced squash and olive oil, then spread onto a rimmed cookie sheet. Bake until squash is soft and start to turn brown (between 20 to 30min.) Remove and set aside. Meanwhile, cook pasta according to directions. When done, drain and rinse well with cold water.

Combine squash, drained orzo, spinach, dried cranberries, and gorgonzola in a large bowl and toss with maple vinaigrette.

To make vinaigrette, place syrup, vinegar, mustard, in a small processor on blade and drizzle in olive oil until combined well.

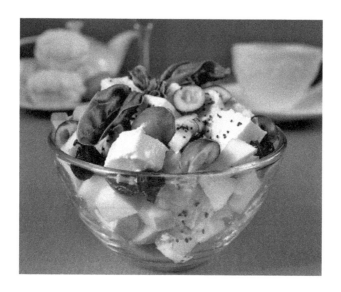

## Harvest Salad

4 slices bacon, diced
2 large eggs
6 cups chopped romaine lettuce
apple, diced
1 pear diced
1/2 cup Fisher nuts pecan halves
1/3 cup fresh cranberries
1/3 cup crumbled goat cheese

For the poppy seed dressing:
1/3 cup mayonnaise
1/4 cup milk

2 tablespoons sugar
1 tablespoon apple cider vinegar
1 tablespoon poppy seeds

To make the poppy seed dressing, whisk together mayonnaise, milk, sugar, apple cider vinegar, and poppy seeds in a small bowl, set aside.

Heat a large skillet over medium high heat. Add bacon and cook until brown and crispy, about 6 to 8 minutes. Transfer to a paper towel-lined plate, set aside.

Place eggs in a pot with boiling water. Cook for 10 minutes. Remove and place in bowl with ice water, until cool off before peeling and dicing.

Place romaine lettuce in a large bowl. Top with arranged rows of bacon, eggs, apple, pear, pecan, cranberries, and goat cheese. Serve with poppy seed dressing.

*There are so many variations of delicious and healthy salads which could help you on your journey toward a healthier lifestyle!*

# Greek Salad

*My family friend owns a Greek restaurant. This is his recipe:*

2 cups of quartered sliced cucumber
1 can of chickpeas drained, rinsed
1 cup of finely diced yellow or red bell pepper
1 1/2 cups of halved cherry tomatoes
1/4 cup minced red onion
1/2 cup of halved olives
1/2 cup crumbled feta cheese
1/4 cup of chopped parsley

Dressing:

1/4 cup olive oil
1 teaspoon Dijon mustard
2 tablespoon red wine vinegar
1 tablespoon lemon juice
1/4 teaspoon garlic powder
1/4 teaspoon onion powder
1/2 teaspoon dried oregano
Some salt and pepper

Dressing:

Combine all of the ingredients in a jar and shake vigorously to mix. Store in the refrigerator.

Salad:

Place the cucumbers, chickpeas, bell pepper, cherry tomatoes, olives, and onion in large bowl. Stir to combine. Add dressing, stir parsley, and sprinkle the feta cheese over the top. Simple but healthy and tasty!

## Soups and Sauces

*Let's look at some delicious and healthy soups and sauces options next!*

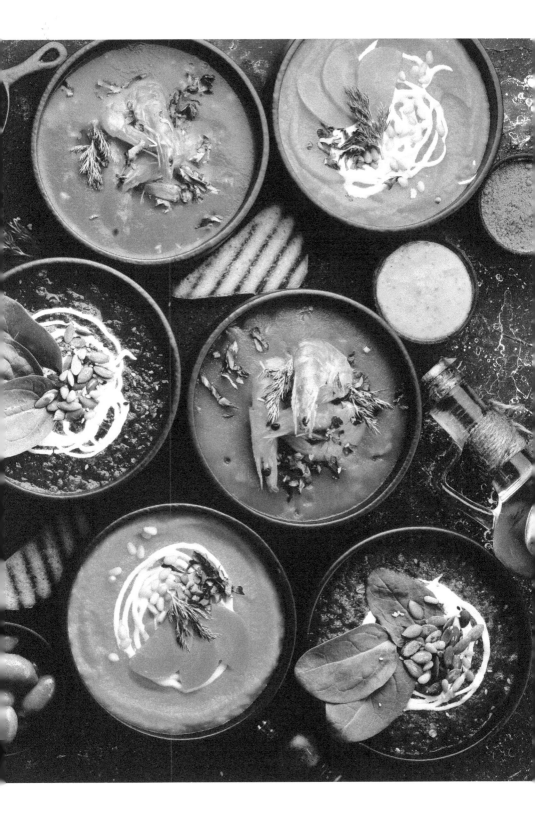

## Black Bean Soup

1 red, yellow, or green sweet pepper, chopped
3/4 cup chopped onion
3/4 cup chopped carrots
2 cloves garlic, minced
3 cups of reduced sodium chicken broth
1 1/2 cups water
2 cans of black beans, rinsed and drained
2 tablespoons snipped fresh cilantro or parsley
1 tablespoon of lemon juice
1 teaspoon dried oregano crushed
1/2 teaspoon black pepper
1/4 cup coconut oil

Spray a large saucepan with nonstick coating. Cook sweet pepper, onion, carrots, and garlic covered in the saucepan over medium-low heat for about five minutes or until tender. Remove from heat. Add broth and water and stir in beans, cilantro, lemon juice, oregano, thyme, chopped red pepper, and black pepper. Place the mixture in a blender. After processing, return the mixture to the saucepan, and bring to a boil. Then reduce the heat and simmer, covered, for ten minutes. It should be ready to eat, but if not, cook a few minutes longer. You may garnish the soup with cilantro and avocado pieces.

## Broccoli Leek Soup

1 tablespoon olive oil
2 medium 350-gram leeks, washed and chopped
4 large cloves of garlic minced
2 large potatoes peeled and cut into cubes
1 large head of broccoli, roughly chopped
4 cups vegetable stock
1 teaspoon sea salt
1 tablespoon lemon juice
1/2 teaspoon oregano or basil

In a large cooking pot, melt the olive oil on a medium heat. When the oil is hot, add leeks and garlic. Sauté for a couple of minutes to soften, stirring often to keep the garlic from burning. Add the potato, broccoli, and stock. Stir and mix in the salt. Cover and let simmer for 15 to 20 minutes until the potatoes and broccoli are fork tender. Remove the pot from the heat. Use an immersion blender to process until you reach your desired consistency. You can also use a blender to puree the soup. Season with more pepper or salt, sprinkling with chopped chives or cheese by choice.

## Broccoli and Turmeric Soup

2 tablespoons butter (vegan butter)
4 cups of leeks chopped
2 tablespoons ginger chopped
8 cups of broccoli florets, roughly 2 heads
1 teaspoon ground turmeric
1 teaspoon salt
Pinch of black pepper
1 tablespoon sesame oil
6 cups chicken stock

Heat a large pan over medium heat and melt the butter. Add the leeks and cook, stirring occasionally, 8 minutes or so until leeks are cooked through. Transfer the leeks to a 5-quart slow cooker with the ginger, broccoli, and turmeric. Cover and cook on low for 3 to 4 hours, until broccoli is tender.

Using a blender, blend until it's creamy and smooth. Serve with yogurt and bread. This soup is anti-inflammatory, so you should definitely try it!

## Summer Squash Soup

2 large sweet onions, chopped
1 medium leek, chopped

2 tablespoons of olive oil
6 garlic cloves, minced
3 medium yellow summer squash, seeded and cubed
4 cups of reduced sodium chicken broth

In a large saucepan, cook onions and leeks in oil until tender. Add garlic and squash and cook for another five to seven minutes. Stir in broth, thyme, and salt. Bring to a boil, reduce heat, cover and simmer for 15 to 20 minutes until squash is tender. When it cools, put it into a blender until smooth. Stir in some lemon juice, and add some pepper.

## Chilled Avocado and Yogurt Soup

2 large firm, ripe avocados
2 1/2 cups buttermilk
1 1/2 cups thick and creamy yogurt
1/4 cup dropped fresh dill
1 tablespoon coarsely chopped fresh mint, plus small mint leaves or
    sprigs.
1 large garlic clove, thinly sliced
1/2 jalapeno chili,
About 1 1/2 tablespoon juice of lemon juice of lemon
About 1 tablespoon sea salt
2 radishes
1 chunk of feta cheese

Half, pit, and peel avocados, and set aside one half. Coarsely chop remaining avocados.

In a blender, whirl buttermilk, yogurt, chopped avocados, dill chopped mint, garlic, and chili until smooth.

Pour soup into a bowl. If you like it thinner, stir in about 1/4 cup cold water. Stir in 1 1/2 tablespoons lemon juice and 1 tablespoon salt. Chill until very cold, 30 minutes. It is must be chilled.

Coarsely shred radishes. Cut reserved half avocado into small dice and sprinkle with a little salt and lemon juice

Taste soup, and add more lemon juice or salt if you like. Ladle into bowls. Place a tuft of radishes and a small spoonful of avocado in center of each serving. Grate a little feta over soup and top with mint leaves.

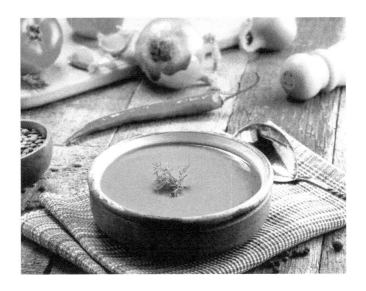

## Creamy Thai Curry Red Lentil Soup

1 tablespoon olive oil
1 medium onion diced
2 cloves garlic sliced
1 tablespoon ginger peeled and diced into small pieces
1 tablespoon Thai red curry paste.
18 ounces sweet potatoes peeled and diced into 1/2-inch cubes
2 medium carrots peeled and diced
3 cups stock (veggie or chicken)
3/4 cup dried red lentils
1 tablespoon fish sauce
1 tablespoon lime juice
1 can coconut milk

*This is delicious soup will give you a little taste of Thailand cuisine!*

Heat olive oil in a large saucepan over medium heat.

Add the onion and cook, stirring occasionally, until translucent and cooked through. Add the garlic and ginger, and cook for a minute. Add the curry paste and cook until onions, garlic, and ginger are coated; and you can smell the curry paste. Add the sweet potato, carrots, stock, lentils, fish sauce, and lime juice.

Cover, bring to a boil, reduce heat, and simmer for 20 minutes until lentils and sweet potato are cooked through.

Using a blender, puree the soup until smooth and creamy. Stir in the coconut milk. Add salt and additional lime juice and fish sauce to taste. Coconut milk, carrots, and ginger make for a zesty change of pace.

## Carrot, Ginger, and Coconut Milk Soup

1 tablespoon coconut oil
1 large white onion, chopped
10 to 12 ounces carrots, peeled and sliced
cloves of garlic
1 tablespoon ginger root, peeled and sliced
1 red chili, seeded and chopped
1 can coconut milk
1 can of vegetable, beef or chicken stock
1 teaspoon cayenne pepper
Pinch of salt and pepper
A few cilantro or basil leaves for garnish

Heat the coconut oil in a large saucepan. And add the chopped onions, garlic, and ginger. Stir for about 3 to 4 minutes until the onions have softened.

Add the carrots and chili cayenne pepper. Give it a quick stir, and allow the flavors to come out while you prepare the liquid ingredients.

Shake the can of coconut milk, and add to the pan, along with your choice of stock. Stir well and bring to the boil, then cover and reduce the heat to a simmer. Simmer for around 20 minutes or until the carrots are soft.

Using a blender, blend the soup until you get the desired creamy consistency. Season to taste, and serve with a few cilantro or basil leaves. This is a filing soup that stands up on its own.

## Roasted Winter Vegetable Soup

Large parsnip, peeled and cubed (1 cup)
3 small sweet potatoes, peeled and diced (2 cups)
1 large carrot, peeled and sliced (1 1/2 cups)
Small celery roots, peeled and diced (1/2 cup)
small onion, diced
1/2 cup celery, finely minced
3 cups of vegetable stock
1 tablespoon fresh rosemary, finely chopped
1 tablespoon herbs (basil, parsley)
1 cup dried baby lima beans
Cloves garlic (minced)
Salt and pepper (to taste)
1 bay leaf

*This is thick soup mostly served in the winter months. The next soup is lighter and normally served in the summertime.*

Preheat the oven to 400 degrees.

Chop root vegetables and toss with 2 tablespoons of oil, half the rosemary and herb, and a dose of salt and pepper. Roast for 20 to 30 minutes, or until everything begins to soften.

In a large dry pot, sauté the onion and celery in the vegetable stock for two minutes. Add the garlic and cook until fragrant.

Add the broth, bean, and remaining herbs. Bring to a boil, cover, and simmer until beans are cooked (about 1 hour). Add more water if necessary.

Add the roasted vegetables, adjust the seasoning, and continue cooking until everything is tender.

## Summer Chicken and Rice Soup

1 pound chicken breasts
28 ounce can crushed tomatoes
10 to 12 ounces carrots, peeled and chopped
4 stalks celery, chopped
4 cloves and minced garlic
1/2 cup rice
4 cups chicken broth
1 tablespoons olive oil
1 teaspoon each basil and oregano
1/2 teaspoon each garlic and onion powder
1/2 teaspoon of salt
2 zucchinis cut into small pieces

Toppings:
Parmesan, juice, plain yogurt, fresh herb, ground pepper, etc.

Place everything except the zucchini in the instant pot or pressure cooker. Set to high pressure for 20 minutes. Release the steam.

Shred the chicken. Stir in the zucchini. Set to high pressure for another 5 minutes. Release the steam. Let the soup rest for a few minutes—it thickens up a bit as it cools.

# Tomato Soup

*No soup list would be complete without some type of tomato soup, so let's make one!*

2 spoons of ghee butter
2 carrots, chopped
Half of a yellow onion, chopped
Cloves of garlic, minced
1 1/2 tablespoons tomato paste
2 tablespoon flour
4 cups chicken broth
1/2 teaspoon of dried thyme
1 bay leaf
28-ounce can of whole tomatoes

*You will want to stock up a bit on your spices so you can prepare these mouth-watering soups in less than a half hour.*

In a large soup pot, put in butter, heat in low heat until melts. Add the carrots, onion, and garlic to the pan. Sauté for 5 to 10 minutes until the vegetables are very aromatic and tender.

Add the tomato paste. Stir for a few minutes until you can see and smell the tomato starting to brown and caramelize. Add the flour, and stir a minute or so.

Pour the tomatoes and their juice into a bowl and crush them with your hands. Add the broth, thyme, bay leaf, and tomatoes to the soup pot. Puree and return to the pot. Add cream if you want to.

# Classic French Onion Soup

3 tablespoons olive oil
1 tablespoon butter
cups thinly sliced onions (about 3 pounds)

3 garlic cloves, minced
2 cartons of beef broth (32 ounces each)
1/2 cup port wine
1/2 teaspoon pepper
1/4 teaspoon salt
24 slices of French bread baguette (1/2 inch thick)
2 large garlic cloves, peeled and halved
3/4 cup Swiss cheese

In an oven, heat 2 tablespoons of oil over medium heat. Add onions, cook and stir until softened for 10 to 13 minutes. Reduce heat to medium-low, cook, stirring occasionally, until deep golden brown for 30 to 40 minutes. Add minced garlic, and cook 2 minutes longer. Stir in wine. Bring to a boil. Cook until the liquid is reduced by half. Add broth, pepper, and salt. Return to a boil. Then reduce heat. Simmer, cover, and stir occasionally for 1 hour. Preheat oven to 400 degrees Fahrenheit. Place baguette slices on a baking sheet, brushed with the remaining oil. Bake until toasted for 3 to 5 minutes on each side. Rub toast with halved garlic.

To serve, place twelve 8-ounce broiler-safe bowls or ramekins on baking sheets. Place two pieces of toast in each. Ladle with soup, top with Swiss cheese. Broil until cheese is melted.

## Onion and Garlic Vegetable Soup

1 tablespoon olive oil
1 large onion, chopped
4 to 6 cloves of garlic, minced
1/4 cup of dry red wine
cups of water

Heat the oil in a 2-quart small soup pot. Add the onion and sauté over medium heat until golden. Add the garlic and continue to sauté until the onion browns lightly. Add the water and the wine. Bring to a simmer, then cover and simmer gently over low heat for 30 to 40 minutes. You may leave in the onion or garlic if you wish or strain the stock. Discard solid or puree them, and add to soup for a thicker consistency. This broth may be used as an extra-flavorful soup stock, or as an alternative with a little extra kick, to a basic vegetable stock. It is also a remedy for the common cold.

## Hummus with Sugar Snap Peas and Basil

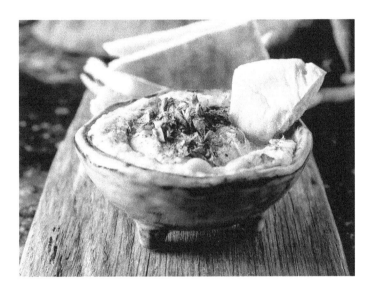

2 cups of thinly sliced sugar snap peas
1 cup lemon juice
1 cup basil leaves
2 tablespoons of white wine vinegar
Kosher salt
2 cups creamy humus with cumin
3 tablespoons of olive oil
2 tablespoons salted, dry-roasted peanuts

Toss peas, basil, and vinegar in a large bowl to combine and season with salt. Spread hummus on a plate, and top with about 1 cup sugar snap peas mixture. Drizzle with oil and top with peanuts.

# Pesto

*Homemade pesto makes for a thoughtful hostess.*

1 cup tightly packed fresh basil
1 cup rightly packed fresh parsley leaves
1 to 2 garlic cloves
1/2 cup olive oil
1/2 cup grated Parmesan cheese
1/4 teaspoon salt

In a food processor, puree all ingredients. Refrigerate for several weeks, or freeze in a tightly covered container. Toss a few tablespoons of pesto with hot-cooked pasta.

# Vegetarian Onion Soup

Tablespoons of extra virgin olive oil
4 large sweet onions, slice
1/2 teaspoon salt
1 teaspoon sugar
2 tablespoons of all-purpose flour
cups mushroom broth
1 tablespoon Worcestershire sauce (vegan)
1/3 cup dry white wine
1/8 teaspoon ground black pepper
1 French baguette
14 ounces of Sincerely Brigitte Tarragon Ginger Cheese

Heat olive oil in a large soup pot. Add onions and salt. Cook over medium heat for 30 minutes. Add 1 teaspoon of sugar and continue cooking for about 50 minutes, stirring frequently. Add flour and mix well. Cook for another 20 minutes. Season the soup with salt and pepper. Add mushroom broth, vegan Worcestershire sauce, and wine. While the soup is cooking, place the cheese in the freezer for

20 minutes. Then shred the cheese, and set aside in the refrigerator. Slice baguette into 1/2-inch pieces. Toast in the broiler till crunchy.

Preheat the oven to 350 degrees Fahrenheit. Line a baking sheet with aluminum foil. Place 4 to 6 oven-proof bowls on the baking sheet and ladle soup into the bowls. Add 3 tablespoons of shredded cheese to each bowl and mix well.

Gently place one or two pieces of bread on top of the soup, and cover the bread with 1/4 cup of cheese per bowl. Place baking sheet in the oven, and bake for 10 minutes. Broil for 1 to 2 minutes, keeping an eye on the bread so that it does not burn. Serve immediately.

# Dinner

*Take a break from meat. Vegetables and grains have protein too!*

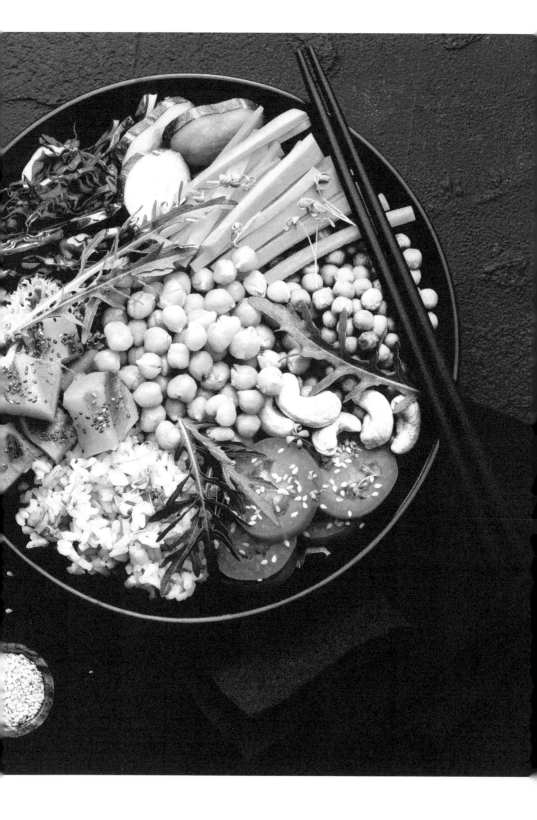

# Lemon Basil Salmon

2 salmon fillets (5 ounces each)
1 tablespoon melted butter
1 tablespoon minced fresh basil
1 tablespoon lemon juice
1/8 teaspoon salt
1/8 teaspoon pepper
Lemon wedges, optional

Prepare campfire or grill for medium heat. Place each fillet, skin side down, on a piece of heavy-duty foil. Mix melted butter, basil, lemon juice, salt, and pepper, spoon over salmon. Fold foil around fish, sealing tightly.

Cook on campfire or in covered grill until fish just begins to flake easily with a fork (about 10 to 15 minutes).

Carefully allow the steam to escape. If desired, serve with lemon wedges.

# Grilled Salmon with Avocado Puree

2 (8-ounce) salmon filets, skin removed
Salt and black pepper, to taste
1 avocado
Lemon juice from 1/2 lemon
1 clove of garlic
1/2 cup fresh basil
1 tablespoon and 1/4 cup olive oil

Season both sides of salmon with salt and pepper. Heat 1 tablespoon olive oil in a skillet over medium-high heat. Add salmon, and sear on both sides for 5 to 6 minutes, or until salmon is cooked to your liking. You can also do this on the grill. While salmon sears, make the avocado sauce. To a food processor or blender, add avocado, lemon juice, garlic, basil, 1/2 cup olive oil, and half and half. Blend until smooth. Taste and season with salt and pepper. Serve salmon with avocado puree on top.

# Eggplant Curry

2 large eggplants, about 1 pound each
3 tablespoons oil
1/2 teaspoon black mustard seeds
1 bunch scallions, finely chopped
4 ounces button mushrooms, halved
2 garlic cloves, minced
1 fresh red chili, finely chopped
1/2 teaspoon chili powder
1 teaspoon ground cumin
1 teaspoon ground coriander
1 teaspoon ground turmeric
1 teaspoon salt
14-ounce can chopped tomato

Brush the eggplants with oil and prick them with a fork. Bake at 400 degrees Fahrenheit for 30 to 35 minutes or until soft. Cut each eggplant in half lengthwise and scoop out the soft flesh into a bowl. Mash the flesh briefly. In a saucepan, put the oil and mustard seeds. Saturate for two minutes. Then add the scallions, mushrooms, garlic, and chili. Cook for five minutes. Stir chili powder, cumin, turmeric, coriander, salt. Cook for three minutes. Add tomatoes and simmer for five minutes. Add the mashed eggplant and cilantro to the saucepan. Bring to a boil and then simmer for five minutes until the sauce thickens. Serve garnished with cilantro sprigs.

## Hibiscus and Shiitake Chipotle Tacos

*Staying on your healthy voyage, you might surprise yourself with these delicious tacos.*

2 tablespoons chipotle-flavored avocado oil
Garlic cloves, finely chopped
1 cup hibiscus, boiled
Shiitake broth (or sub natural veggie broth) to taste
1 cup fresh shiitake
Salt and pepper to taste
Chili flakes to taste
Garlic powder to taste
Onion power to taste
A pinch of monk fruit
Equal amounts of quinoa and cassava flours
Cactus flour (1/4 of the amount of above flours)
Creamy base of your choice: garlic hummus, Greek yogurt
1 avocado

Heat oil in frying pan and cook garlic until golden. Set garlic aside. Cook hibiscus for about 3 minutes, adding broth slowly so it cooks. Add shitake, spices, and monk fruit. Continue to cook while stirring. Add more broth if needed. Add garlic, and cook for 2 more minutes.

To make tortillas, combine cassava and quinoa flours. Mix in cactus flour. Add enough water to make dough and form four balls. Use a tortilla rolling pin or your hands to make even tortillas. Spread creamy base on tortilla, and fill with hibiscus mixture.

Top with avocado.

## Stuffed Zucchini with Chicken

3 medium zucchinis, cut in half lengthwise
1 tablespoon olive oil
2 cups cooked shredded chicken
2 cups tomato sauce
1 cup shredded mozzarella and cheddar cheese
Salt and pepper to taste (optional)
Fresh parsley (chopped)

Cut the edges of the zucchini, and slice each one in half lengthwise. Using a spoon remove the flesh from the center of the zucchini halves. Chop the scooped-out zucchini flesh and set aside.

Pour 1/2 cup of the tomato sauce into a casserole and spread well. Preheat the oven to 375 degrees Fahrenheit. Add olive oil, chicken, and chopped zucchini to a large nonstick skillet. Sauté over medium heat for 3 minutes or until the chopped zucchini is soft. Add tomato pasta sauce and salt and black pepper to taste and cook for few minutes. Stuff the scooped-out zucchini halves with the chicken mixture. Pour the remaining sauce over zucchini, and cover the casserole with aluminum foil.

Bake the zucchini for 30 to 35 min. Remove the casserole from the oven. Add shredded cheese. Bake for more 3 to 5 minutes until cheese is melted. Garnish with parsley!

## Sweet Hidden Veggie Turkey Burgers

*Sometimes we want to eat a lighter meal, and this recipe is perfect for that!*

4 ounces cut baby carrots
1/4 sweet white onion, finely chopped
16 ounces lean ground turkey
1 tablespoon pure maple syrup
1 tablespoon whole grain mustard
2 teaspoons minced garlic
1 teaspoon sea salt
1/2 teaspoon paprika
2 ounces of white or yellow shredded cheddar cheese
2 tablespoons extra virgin olive oil
Eggs, cooked

Chop baby carrots, and place into a food processor. Process until very finely shredded.

Spray small skillet with cooking spray and cook onions until soft. Pour all ingredients, including shredded carrots, onions, and excluding eggs, into a large mixing bowl and combine well using hands or a hand mixer on low speed.

Separate the mixture into four equal portions and form into burgers. Wrap the burgers individually, and store in the fridge for 15 to 30 minutes to set.

Preheat a cast iron skillet or grill. Place the burgers, and cook 3 to 4 minutes per side until cooked through.

Top each burger with egg.

## Green Bean Casserole

12 ounces frozen French-style green beans, steamed
1 tablespoon coconut oil
8 ounces sliced white mushrooms, finely chopped
1/4 cup finely diced white onion.
3 tablespoons coconut flour.
1 cup chicken broth
1/2 cup milk

For the topping:
1 tablespoon coconut oil
1/2 cup finely diced white onion
2 slices sandwich bread of your choice
2 tablespoons shredded Parmesan cheese
Salt and pepper to taste

Preheat oven to 350 degrees Fahrenheit.

Spray a medium saucepan liberally with cooking spray, then warm over medium heat. Add 1/4 cup finely diced white onion and mushrooms, and sauté until onions are translucent and liquid has released from mushrooms. Sprinkle onion/mushroom mixture with coconut flour, stirring in one teaspoon at a time until each is incorporated.

Add vegetable broth and milk. Stir well to combine, and bring to a gentle rolling boil. Reduce heat and simmer, stirring occasionally until the mixture has thickened or reduced by about half.

Reduce two slices of bread to crumbs using a food processor. Add Parmesan cheese, and pulse again until well blended.

Spray a medium skillet liberally with cooking spray, then warm over medium heat. Add 1/2 cup finely diced white onion, and sauté until translucent.

Sprinkle onions with bread crumb-and-cheese mixture, stirring in a little bit at a time until everything is incorporated. Sauté until everything is a rich, golden brown.

## Spinach and Zucchini Lasagna

1 tablespoon extra-virgin olive oil
1/2 onion (finely chopped)
4 garlic cloves (crushed)
2 tablespoons tomato paste
1 28-ounce can crushed tomatoes with the juice or 1 3/4 pound of fresh tomatoes (peeled, seeded, and diced)
Salt and ground fresh black pepper to taste
1 tablespoon chopped fresh basil
3 cups spinach
15 ounces part skim ricotta
1 large egg
1/2 cup freshly grated Parmesan cheese
4 medium zucchinis (sliced 1/8 thick)
16 ounces part-skim mozzarella cheese (shredded)
1/2 tablespoon parsley (chopped)

In a saucepan, heat olive oil medium heat. Add onions, and cook 4 to 5 minutes until they are soft and golden. Add garlic and sauté, being careful not to burn. Add tomato paste, and stir well. Add crushed tomatoes, including the juice in case you are using tomato cans. Add salt and ground fresh black pepper. Cover and bring to a low simmer for 25 to 30 minutes. Finally, remove from the heat. And add fresh basil, spinach, and stir well. Adjust the seasoning if you think it is necessary.

Preheat oven to 375 degrees Fahrenheit. Arrange the zucchini slices in a single layer on a baking sheet, and coat it with cooking oil spray. Put in oven for 15 minutes. Remove from the oven. Wait about 5 minutes to remove any excess moisture with paper towels if you think it is necessary.

In a medium-sized bowl, mix ricotta cheese, Parmesan cheese, and an egg. Stir well.

In a casserole dish, spread some tomato sauce on the bottom. Layer 5 or 6 zucchini slices to cover. Place some of the ricotta cheese mixture and top the mozzarella cheese. Repeat the layers until all your ingredients are used up. Top with sauce and mozzarella.

Cover the casserole dish with aluminum foil, and bake for 30 minutes covered and 10 to 15 minutes uncovered. Let it sit for about 10 minutes before serving garnish with parsley.

## Confetti Vegetable Risotto

1 cup chopped mushrooms
1/2 cup chopped carrots
1/2 cup chopped zucchini
1 clove garlic, minced
2 tablespoons olive oil
1 cup long grain rice
1/2 cup frozen corn

1/2 cup frozen peas
1 1/2 cup reduced sodium chicken broth
1 1/2 cups water
3/4 teaspoon dried basil, crushed
1/4 teaspoon dried thyme, crushed
1/8 teaspoon pepper
3/4 cup grated Parmesan cheese

Confetti vegetable risotto is not easy to make. In a large saucepan, cook mushrooms, carrots, zucchini, and garlic in hot oil for a few minutes. Stir in rice, peas, corn, and cook for three minutes. In another saucepan, combine broth, water, basil, thyme, and pepper. Bring to boil. Add one cup of the boiling broth mixture to the rice mixture. Cook over medium heat, stirring constantly until nearly all liquid has been absorbed. Add more broth mixture to cover the rice, stirring constantly until that portion has been absorbed. Continue this until all liquid is gone, and rice is tender. This takes about 25 minutes. Remove from heat. Stir in Parmesan cheese and serve.

## Desserts

*Desserts don't need to be unhealthy. Give yourself a treat while eating healthy at the same time. Bon appétit!*

# Overnight Chia Pudding

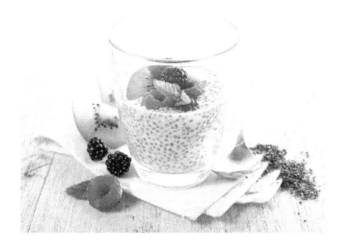

1/2 chia seeds
2 1/2 cups almond milk
1/4 cup toasted coconut
1/4 cup toasted pecans
Tablespoons maple syrup

In a 350 degrees Fahrenheit oven, toast the coconut and pecans on a baking sheet until the coconut begins to turn golden brown. Set aside and allow to cool.

In a medium sized bowl, mix the chia seeds, coconut, and pecans together. Add the almond milk to the bowl and stir. Wrap the bowl in foil, and put into the fridge overnight.

In the morning, drizzle the pudding with a little maple syrup, and enjoy!

## Coconut with Almond and Cashew Chews (No Bake)

1 1/2 cups raw almonds
1 1/2 cup raw cashews

2 tablespoons tahini sesame butter
1 tablespoon flaxseeds ground
1 1/2 cup unsweetened coconut
3/4 cup honey
1 tablespoon vanilla extract
3/4 teaspoon sea salt

Place almonds and cashews in a food processor and pulse until finely chopped. Add flax, honey, tahini, vanilla, coconut, and salt, and pulse a few more times

Press firmly into 9-by-5-by-1-inch pan and refrigerate for several hours. Cut into small squares (or roll into little balls), and store in air tight container in refrigerator. Remove just before serving.

## Cranberry Oat Breakfast Cookies (Gluten-Free)

1 1/2 cups blanched almond flour
1/4 cup coconut flour
1/4 cup coconut sugar
1 teaspoon cinnamon
1/2 teaspoon nutmeg
1/2 teaspoon baking soda
Pinch of salt
1 cup rolled oats
1/2 cup dried cranberries
1 egg
1/2 cup butter, melted
1/4 cup maple syrup
1/3 cup applesauce
Teaspoon vanilla extract

Preheat oven to 350 degrees Fahrenheit and line two sheet pans with parchment paper.

Put dry ingredients into a medium-sized bowl, and stir together with a large spoon, breaking up any flour or cranberry clumps as you go.

Whisk the egg, maple syrup, applesauce, and vanilla together in a small bowl with a fork.

Add the butter and applesauce mixture to the dry ingredients, and stir until the dough becomes nice.

Scoop dough by the spoon, and put onto a pan. Bake cookies for 12 minutes. Cool cookies for a few minutes on the pan, then transfer to a wire rack to cool completely.

## Gluten-Free Yogurt Banana Bread (1 Loaf)

*Keeping with the gluten-free theme, here is another good choice:*

2 very ripe bananas
1/2 cup natural yogurt
Tablespoons melted coconut oil
3 tablespoons honey
2/3 cup rice flour
1/3 cup ground almonds
1/2 teaspoon baking soda
1 teaspoon cinnamon
Pinch of salt

Pre-heat the oven at 325 degrees Fahrenheit, and line a 9-inch loaf tin with baking paper.

Mash the bananas in a bowl. If your bananas are not ripe enough yet, you can put them in the oven for few minutes until the skins brown. Then wait for them to cool before mashing. Add the yogurt, eggs, melted coconut oil, and honey to the bananas and mix well. Add the dry ingredients, and blend until smooth.

Pour the mixture into loaf tin. Bake for about 40 minutes until knife inserted comes out clean. Cool in the tin. Then use the baking paper to lift it out and transfer to a plate or rack.

## Raspberry Cinnamon Protein Coffee Cake

2 cups old-fashioned oats
2 cups low-fat cottage cheese
Whole eggs or two cups liquid egg whites
1 tablespoon vanilla extract
2/3 cup brown sugar
1/4 teaspoon liquid stevia
1 teaspoon cinnamon
1/4 teaspoon nutmeg
1 tablespoon plus 1 teaspoon baking powder
1 1/2 cups frozen raspberries

Preheat oven to 350 degrees Fahrenheit. Spray pan with coconut oil baking spray.

In a blender or food processor, blend oats until they form fine flour. Add remaining ingredients (except for raspberries), and blend on high for 1 minute or until a batter forms.

Spoon the batter into a prepared pan. Sprinkle raspberries over the top and gently stir into batter with a spoon. Bake the cake for 40 minutes until golden brown and set in the center. Cool completely on a wire rack.

# Lime and Basil Pie

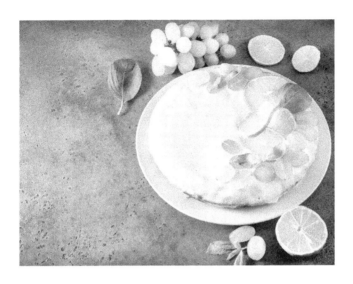

1 package (8 ounces) reduced fat cream cheese
1 can (14 ounces) condensed milk
1 tablespoon grated lime zest
1/2 cup lime juice
2 large egg yolks
1/4 cup minced fresh basil
1 reduced-fat graham cracker crust (8 inches)
Whipped cream

Preheat the oven to 325 degrees Fahrenheit. In a large bowl, beat cream cheese until smooth and gradually beat in milk. Add lime zest, juice, and egg yolks. Beat just until blended. Stir in basil. Pour into crust. Bake 15 to 18 minutes or until center is set. Cool one hour on a wire rack. Refrigerate at least two hours before serving. If desired, serve with whipped cream and fruits of your liking.

# Spicy Pumpkin Seeds

*Not a lover of sweets? How about a salty and spicy snack instead?*

(Serves 6 to 8 people)
1 tablespoon coconut oil
1 pound of raw pumpkin seeds
1/2 teaspoon cayenne pepper
Teaspoons of Tabasco sauce

Heat the oil in a large pan over medium heat. Add pumpkin seeds, and sauté for two to three minutes until they pop and turn golden brown. Add cayenne and Tabasco, toss, and continue to cook for another two minutes. Transfer to a sheet tray and carefully spread the seeds out in a single layer, and set aside to cool before serving. Enjoy!

# Roasted Red Onion Flowers

Red medium onions or sweet onions with roots
Tablespoons of olive oil
Salt (smoked salt is delicious)
A sprig of rosemary or some bay leaves
Freshly ground pepper

Preheat oven to 350 degrees Fahrenheit. Cut onions into eight pieces. Drizzle olive oil into a baking dish. Arrange onions root end down. Roast for 40 minutes. Then add more olive oil, and roast another 20 minutes. Season with salt and pepper and serve.

# Chapter 7

# Natural Healing Plants and Home Remedies

Natural healing started from the idea that food and vitamins can be your best medicine. You can help yourself, your family, and friends to get even healthier!

Most medical histories chronicle great achievements by great men: Hippocrates, the father of medicine; Galen, Rome's leading physician; William Harvey, the discoverer of blood circulation; Edward Jenner's inoculations against smallpox; Louis Pasteur's germ theory; and Alexander Fleming's discovery of penicillin. Yes, the contributions of these men have changed the world. However, the reality is that many medically untrained women still provide the majority of the world's primary care. Women healers have been called green women, witches, old wives, or nurses. Most physicians have never taken women's folk wisdom seriously and dubbed them old wives' tales. The medical profession promotes the ideas that family doctors are our primary providers, but studies show that before people call health professionals, about 90 percent consult a friend or family member. The informal health advisors are almost always women. After many stressful situations, I had a gallbladder attack and had to stay in the hospital for a few days. I was forty years old at the time and lived in my birth country of Lithuania. The physician in charge of the clinic told me, "I am an excellent doctor and will give you the best service, but you are an agronomist and work with plants. Try healing yourself with plants. This will be the best choice for you." It was the best advice I ever received. After my agronomy studies, I became an alternative medicine consultant. I know plants have healing power and can save many lives. Plants continue to be a major source of medicine, as they have been used throughout human history. The growing population of developing countries with few medical professionals continue to rely heavily on the use of traditional medicine as their primary source of health care. Medicinal plants are now being given serious attention by mainstream medical science.

Michael J. Balick, PhD, vice president for botanical science, director and philecology curator of Institute of Economic Botany, The New York Botanical Garden, explains: "Mother Nature is a brilliant chemist. From earliest times our ancestors have learned to use real value for improving our lives." He goes on to say, "I always suggest that anything taken as medicine—be it a product or an herbal supplement or tea, can be used under the supervision of a knowledgeable professional to ensure an optimum result." I would like to share information about some plants from my organic garden. It might surprise you how beneficial they can be for your health!

## Cayenne Pepper

The first written appearance of cayenne to history books was in 1493 when Peter Martyn wrote of its arrival in Italy after Columbus's voyage. Discovery of cayenne was important because of the growing European interest in and the market for herbs. Cayenne was probably cultivated for hundreds of years in the tropical Americas, Africa, India, and other tropical areas of the world. Jethro Kloss, the twentieth century American herbalist, called cayenne "one of the most wonderful herb medicines that we have," and he termed it a "specific" for fevers. "Take some in capsules, followed by a glass of water," he said. The active ingredient in cayenne pepper is a substance called capsaicin, which when taken internally or applied externally, acts as a powerful stimulant. Hot and stimulating, cayenne peppers are like a jump-start for a cold engine on a frosty morning. It brings welcome new life back to muscles and gets your heart beating faster, increasing the flow of blood all throughout the body. The heat of cayenne warms up stiff arthritic joints and relaxes away back pain. The longer you use it, the better it works.

The Cancer Treatment Center of America listed eleven foods with cancer-fighting properties and cayenne is near the top. There are reasons for that. A single teaspoon of cayenne pepper imparts 15 percent of the daily recommended value in vitamin A and 3 percent of the vitamin E. It is also an excellent source of vitamin C, which provides collagen synthesis to retain healthy skin, blood vessels, bones, and organs and helps boost your immunity. It is a good source of vitamin B6, manganese, niacin, and riboflavin. Cayenne is an extremely effective treatment for heart and blood circulation problems.

It's a miracle for congestive heart failure and beneficial for someone who has circulatory problems, such as high or low blood pressure, elevated cholesterol, high triglycerides, and even varicose veins. An impressive number of other health benefits can be gleaned by ingesting careful amounts of cayenne pepper, especially in regard to capsaicin for pain relief. In fact, capsaicin is now widely known in medical circles as a useful treatment, even for painful, debilitating arthritis. Studies also indicate that cayenne pepper clears congestion. It should not come as a surprise that the heat from cayenne pepper can help loosen up phlegm and mucus in your longs and nasal passages so that you can be rid of it. It also reduces headache pain, fights inflammation, helps stop the spread of prostate cancer, lowers the risk of type 2 diabetes, and aids in weight loss. Studies have shown that a compound in cayenne effectively suppressed the development of fungal strains while remaining nontoxic to animal cells. Cayenne is also a well-known digestive aid and stimulates the flow of enzyme production and gastric juice. It even can get rid of intestinal gas.

# Garlic

Garlic may be the best example of the continuum between plants as food and plants as medicine. One of the most ancient remedies known to humanity, garlic is a staple in the diets of an incredibly diverse number of cultures. Garlic was once thought to possess magical power against evil and was widely used in charms and spells. Many of the legends surrounding it has to do with strength, speed, and endurance. Egyptian slaves ate garlic as they built the pyramids. The Israelites nibbled it before their escape from Egypt and later longed for the herb during their wilderness wanderings. European legend says that if a man chews on a garlic bulb during a foot race, no one will be able to get ahead of him.

Medicinally, garlic has been prescribed since pre-biblical times. Ancient herbalists in the Far East, used it in the calendar which dates back to 2000 BC. An Egyptian medical listing of 1550 BC recommends garlic as a remedy for twenty-two problems including headaches, worms, tumors, and heart ailments. Southern Europeans also used it in folk medicines, as well as their foods.

Active constituents in garlic

The sulfur compound allicin is produced by crushing or chewing of the fresh bulb of garlic. Allicin produces other sulfur compounds, including allyl sulfides, ajoene, and vinyldithiins. These compounds are found only in garlic oil products by maceration (not in steam-distilled garlic). One common use of garlic includes the reduction of cholesterol and triglyceride levels. These conditions lead to poor circulation and even obstructions of blood vessels. More than 250 publications have shown that garlic effectively lowers cholesterol and triglycerides. Garlic interferes with the creation of cholesterol in the liver.

Few more uses of garlic:

*Reducing blood pressure.* In the book *Herbal Prescriptions for Better Health: Your Up-to-Date Guide to the Most Effective Herbal Treatments* written by N. D. Donald J. Brown, it says, "Garlic is one part of an overall program for lowering mildly elevated blood pressure, and is not a substitute for stronger blood pressure medications."

*Curing infections.* Herbalists have long claimed that garlic was a good germ killer. In India, garlic is used to wash wounds and ulcers. During World War I, army doctors daubed garlic juice on sterilized sphagnum moss and applied it to infected wounds. Experiments have shown that garlic is effective against some influenza viruses, fungi, and yeast, such as the one that causes athlete's foot. Ear infections can be helped with wrapping one garlic clove in tissue and inserted into the ear overnight. Pain is almost immediately gone, and the infection starts to clear up.

*Respiratory ailments.* In traditional medicine of both China and Europe, garlic is recommended for tuberculosis by treating patients with an inhalant of garlic oil or juice. It is also recommended to take a teaspoon of garlic syrup for coughs.

*Curing for worms and other parasites.* An old wife's remedy for pinworms was an enema of raw garlic. Raw garlic also works well on rashes and bug bites. It stops the itching immediately.

*Coughing.* Coughs can be soothed with the juice of 8 to 10 garlic cloves mixed with 2 tablespoons of honey, used four times a day. Tonsilitis can be cured with boiling a garlic clove for a couple of minutes in one and a half cup of water and then add a pinch of salt, a teaspoon of butter, and a pinch of pepper. Sprinkle some nutmeg over the liquid and drink.

*Asthma.* Asthma can be aided with syrup of garlic bulbs made by boiling the garlic and adding an equal amount of vinegar and then some sugar. Each morning, eat a bulb of garlic and a spoonful of the garlic syrup.

*Memory.* Older adults often have problems with memory, but garlic can keep you mentally nimble. Eleanor Roosevelt, who was renowned for her excellent memory, said it was due to eating three cloves of garlic a day. She would dip them in chocolate or honey.

*Nosebleeds.* Herbal physicians would use a paste made from crushed garlic for nosebleeds. You don't put it in your nose. You place it on the bottom of your foot. Use a circle of garlic paste about the size of a half dollar on the foot that is on the same side as your nosebleed.

*Poison ivy.* Garlic can be used to cure the itch of poison ivy. Boil four cloves of garlic in a cup of water, and apply it with a clean cloth to the affected area. Repeat until itching stops.

*Sinus infections.* Sinus infections can be cured with ten drops of clear garlic juice mixed with water applied to each nostril three times a day for three days.

*Vaginal itching.* Vaginal itching can be cured with an application of six cloves of garlic sliced and added to just boiled water. After the mixture steeps for twenty minutes, strain and apply it to the genital area, and use it as a douche. The itching should disappear in no time.

*Garlic as a natural antibacterial.* The little bulb doesn't stop at just those cures. It is particularly effective in treating upper respiratory viral infections due to is immune-enhancing properties and its ability to clear mucus from the lungs. It destroys and inhibits various bacteria and fungi, with an antibacterial action equivalent to 1 percent penicillin. Garlic benefits for men and women also include it being an effective ally against strep, staph, and even anthrax bacteria. Garlic is the only antibiotic that can actually kill anthrax bacteria and protect the body from the poisons that are causing the infection. It is known that the most sensitive bacterium to garlic is the deadly Bacillus anthracis, which produces the poison anthrax. Even the forefather of medicine, Louis Pasteur acknowledged garlic to be as effective as penicillin, and late studies showed similar activity to a more modern antibiotic, chloramphenicol. In a Japanese journal, *Journal of Nutritional Science and Vitaminology*, 2003 August, 49(4):297–9, "Bacteriocidal Activity of Garlic Powder Against Bacillus Anthracis," concluded, "A 1% water solution of garlic powder in the test tube method killed B. anthracis at 10(7) cfu/mL within 3 h of treatment at room temperature." Garlic is among the few herbs that have universal usage and recognition. Its daily use aids and supports the body in ways that no other herb does! According to a survey of people that lived to be 100 years or older, garlic is the key to a long life. Indian nutritionist, Dr. Lai Narain of New Delhi's College of Public Health, found that 98 percent if these centenarians ate at least one garlic clove per day. The many uses of garlic make it an herbal miracle!

## Aloe Vera (Syn: Aloe barbadensis)

One of the first mentions of aloe vera appears in the Papyrus Ebers around 1550. It is widely believed that Egyptian queens Nefertiti and Cleopatra used aloe vera every day to preserve their beauty. Egypt was not the only a part of the world that found value in aloe vera. Records from as early as the seventeenth century show that East India Trading Company relied heavily on aloe for its commercial value. With such amazing historical uses, aloe vera has earned nicknames from around the globe, names like the "silent healer," "burn plant," and "first aid plant." The part of the aloe vera that is used is the inner leaf. The 75 constituents of aloe vera include enzymes, sugars, lignin, saponins, salicylic acids, and amino acids. It is rich in vitamin D, A, C, and E. It has calcium, copper, zinc, chromium, selenium, sodium, potassium, magnesium, and manganese. The leaf juices of the aloe plant have many important medical uses and are put in many gels, creams, and lotions.

Immune system

Aloe vera supports the immune system, support nutrient absorption from the gut, and this includes iron absorption. Iron carries free oxygen molecules from lung to all over the body. Aloe vera helps maintain blood-oxygen levels. Aloe helps absorb nutrients by keeping the digestive tract clear of debris through bowel regularity.

Digestion

Aloe vera helps support normal digestion. It contains two enzymes that help normal digestion: amylase and lipase. The plant also keeps stomach acid levels balanced to support a normal gut environment. Aloe vera eases digestive discomfort. Common digestive concerns such as gas, diarrhea, constipation, and abdominal pain affect a lot of people; for that, aloe vera may be able to help. Studies show decreased gas, bloating, and discomfort in those who take regular aloe supplements.

Vitamins

Aloe vera is rich in vitamins, minerals, and antioxidants. This includes vitamin A (beta-carotene), which is important for healthy skin, teeth, bones, and eyes, also vitamin C which is essential for metabolism, skin health, and immune function, and last but not least, vitamin E which protects the skin from UV damage.

Aloe eye drops

Neville Baron, MD, an ophthalmologist in Secaucus, New Jersey, has found evidence that an aloe extract absorbs damaging ultraviolet rays, and he suggests that aloe may be the source of the "miracle eye drop of the twentieth century." Aloe vera eye drops may help people with cataracts, degeneration of the retina, or abnormalities of the lens. Those with normal eyes may be protected from ultraviolet damage by using them.

Aloe and hydrogen peroxide spray

You can make an aloe spray for easing the pain of soar areas. Pour aloe vera juice into a bowl, and add one cup of 1.5 percent hydrogen peroxide solution. Mix and pour into a bottle with a spray nozzle. Apply to sore joints, elbows, knees, neck, and feet. Massage it in. You can apply it one to three times a day to ease the pain of certain areas.

Aloe vera juice

This juice strengthens immunity and protects the cells from being penetrated by bacteria and viruses. It directly stimulates the immune system. It treats intestinal ailments. The properties in aloe vera juice make it an effective remedy for digestive ailments. It can soothe a nervous stomach, neutralize excess gastric acids, and eliminate harmful intestinal bacteria, allowing intestinal flora to regenerate.

Aloe vera juice has tissue-restoring properties and is antibacterial. It cleans and detoxifies the body, and when used as part of a purification regimen, it can be beneficial with fasting or cleansing diets that eliminate intestinal toxins. Drinking three to four ounces of aloe vera juice daily before meals either by itself or mixed with fruit juice can prevent colds and flu. For children, limit the aloe vera to one tablespoon three times a day. Aloe vera juice can be applied directly to a burn to relieve pain and cool the skin. Aloe encourages the skin to regenerate and prevents the wound from becoming infected. Dip a sterile cloth in aloe vera juice and place it on the burned area. Change the dressing several times a day. You can also use the juice in a spray bottle and spray the affected area several times a day. For deep burns or those that cover a large area, always see a health care provider. For colds, drink a half of a cup for fresh aloe vera with five tablespoons of honey and fresh lemon juice. Do this three times a day. Aloe vera can also be used in a mouthwash to help gum inflammation.

However, don't use aloe vera if you have any allergies to the Liliaceae family (garlic, onions, and tulips), if you are pregnant, have a cardiac disease, low blood sugar, or are taking medication. Always check with your physician first.

## Echinacea

For a time, echinacea enjoyed official status as a result of being listed in the US National Formulary from 1916–1950. However, the use of echinacea fell out of favor in the United States with the discovery of antibiotics. But now people are becoming interested in echinacea again because some antibiotics don't work as well as they used to against certain bacteria. It has been used by Native Americans for hundreds of years as a pain killer. Echinacea is used to fight infections from colds, flu, and other respiratory illnesses, urinary tract infections, earaches, tonsillitis, and streptococcus infections. Commercially it is available as tablets, juice, and tea. There are concerns about the quality of the product. They are frequently mislabeled, and some may not even contain echinacea, one of the most effective and popular herbal remedies for strengthening the immune system, which may mobilize immune system cells and stimulate their disease-fighting activity. The components of echinacea are from its two main active ingredients echinacosides in the flower and root and polysaccharide heteroxylan in the leaves. There are nine varieties of echinacea, but only the purple coneflower or *Echinacea purpurea* is considered a remedy. Some use it to treat fever blisters. Place a few drops of pressed echinacea juice on a cotton swab or ball and gently apply it to the affected area. This easy home remedy can halt the progression of the lesion or even prevent them outright. Others use it to treat sore throats, urinary tract infections, and vaginal yeast infections.

The University of Connecticut did a research and concluded that echinacea reduces the duration of the common cold by almost one and a half days and reduces the chance of catching the common cold by 58 percent. The *FASEB Journal* published a study in 2016 "Chicoric Acid Supplementation Prevents Systemic Inflammation-Induced Memory Impairment and Amyloidogenesis via Inhibition of NF-$x$B" and concluded that echinacea demonstrated inflammatory mediators and might prove useful in the treatment of Alzheimer's disease. *Phytotherapy Research* published "The potential use of Echinacea in Acne: Control of Propionibacterium Acnes Growth and Inflammation" in 2010. It concluded that echinacea could treat acne due to its ability to kill bacteria and reduce inflammation. A 2015 *Journal of Ethnopharmacology*, "Echinacea Complex-Chemical View and Anti-Asthmatic Profile" concluded that echinacea was a good supplement for the treatment of asthma.

Recommendations for use of echinacea

Echinacea is available over the counter in many health food stores and pharmacies. There are so many different forms including liquid extracts, capsules, pills, and echinacea tea. There is no formal proof on how to best use echinacea. Some sources claim that it is most effective when taken as soon as the symptoms occur and to use it for seven to ten days. Remember to use an alcohol-free preparation.

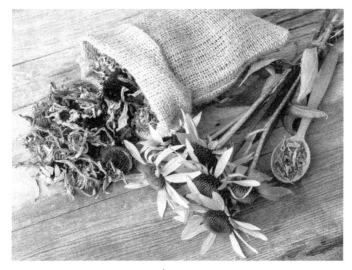

Echinacea.

As a final note of caution, the *Archives of Internal Medicine* reports the results of a study that took eleven brands of echinacea and discovered that only four of them actually contained what was on their label. Ten percent had no echinacea at all, and half of the products did not contain the labeled amount of ingredients. To ensure that you receive the most echinacea benefits, always purchase from a trusted brand. Discuss the use of echinacea with your doctor and ask which brand you should use.

# Ginger

Ancient writing from Rome, Greece, China, and Arab countries all describe ginger's uses as a medicine. It was especially used as a treatment for stomach issues, including nausea and diarrhea. Other traditional medical uses include using ginger for treating muscles and joint pain, cold and flu symptoms, stomach pain, menstrual cramps, and skin burns. One tablespoon of ginger contains 4.8 calories, 1.07 grams of carbohydrates, 12 grams of dietary fiber, 0.5 grams of protein, 0.5 grams of fat, and 0.1 gram of sugar. It also contains vitamin B3, B6, iron, potassium, vitamin C, zinc, niacin, folate, and riboflavin. Ginger contains more than four hundred chemical compounds that have antioxidant and anti-inflammatory properties that can help the body in a variety of different ways.

Ginger has been recommended for colds and flu. *The Journal of Ethnopharmacology* in January of 2013 concluded that fresh ginger has anti-viral properties. One way that ginger helps is that it is a diaphoretic (meaning that ginger causes sweating). German scientists studied sweating and concluded it creates a protein they called dermcidin that kills bacteria. Fresh ginger also stimulates mucosal cells to produce beta-interferon to kill viruses.

Ginger has been proven to help relieve pain. The University of Georgia did a story that found a daily dose of ginger reduced exercise-induced pain by 25 percent. A study published in Pain Medicine in 2015 suggested that drinking ginger tea helped block the body's production of prostaglandins that are the cause of dysmenorrhea. Another study from Pain Medicine in 2016 concluded that ginger even helped with heavy bleeding. Ginger has also some use in lowering blood sugar. In the *Iranian Journal of Pharmaceutical Research* (winter of 2015), "Ginger supplementation significantly reduced the levels of fasting blood sugar." They concluded that more studies need to be done with a larger number of patients and a longer study period. In the *International Journal of Food Sciences and Nutrition* in 2014 had an article called "The Effect of Ginger Consumption of Glycemic Status, Lipid Profile, and Some Inflammatory Markers in Patients with Type 2 Diabetes Mellitus." The study concluded that ginger improved insulin sensitivity. It also reduced triglycerides and total cholesterol. Ginger may also help treat a wide range of cancers including breast cancer. The March 11, 2015, issue of the *Journal of Agricultural Food Chemistry* says that one of the components of ginger, 6-shagoal, targets breast cancer without causing harm to the body. Other studies showed that ginger was effective in treating lung cancer in mice. They concluded that compounds in ginger could be as "much as 10,000 times more effective in chemotherapy in targeting the root cause of cancer.

Many cultures have discovered how good ginger is for curing nausea. Modern medicine concurs. In the March 31, 2016, *Integrative Medicine Insights*, the article, "The Effectiveness of Ginger in the Prevention of Nausea and Vomiting during Pregnancy and Chemotherapy" by Inaki Lete and Jose Allue, concluded ginger was safe and effective to treat nausea and vomiting during pregnancy. They also concluded that ginger would aid those going through chemotherapy. Roy Altman, MD, formerly of the University of Miami, and now University of California Los Angeles says, "Research shows that ginger affects certain inflammatory processes at a cellular level." He was part of a study comparing ginger to NSAIDS. The study concluded that ginger reduced stiffness in knee joints by 40 percent over the placebo.

## Basil

A medical herb, as well as a sweet pungent culinary seasoning, basil is native to India but is now grown in temperate regions all over the world. Basil is one of the most familiar herbs because it is widely used in Italian cuisine, particularly in tomato-based dishes. But it also complements many other foods, including meat, poultry, salads, and soups. It can also be used in certain desserts. Thanks to its antispasmodic properties, basil is used for treating flatulence and upset stomachs. It also helps ease tension and reduce sleep. Its pungent taste triggers the production of saliva, enabling the body to digest food more effectively. It further aids digestion by increasing appetite and the flow of bile. Basil can stimulate the chill in the nose, helping to clear the nasal passages of mucus and disease-causing bacteria.

Components of basil

The therapeutic action of the herb, basil, is due to its essential oils, primarily methyl chavicol. Fresh basil contains carotenoids and folic acid. In its dried form, basil is a good source of calcium, potassium, and iron.

Basil for the kitchen

To store fresh leaves, wrap them in paper towels, and place them in plastic bags in the refrigerator. For longer storage, put the bags in a container, cover them with olive oil, and refrigerate for ten to fourteen days. If you need to store them longer, you should freeze them: puree them in a blender or food processor. Then place the puree in an ice cube tray and add a little water to cover. Or you could dry the basil in a tightly closed container in a dark place at the room temperature. This prevents flavor loss. Basil wine is a digestive aid. Steep a small bunch of fresh basil in a bottle of white wine for twenty-four hours. Then strain the wine and refrigerate. Drink a four-ounce glass after meals. Basil tea can soothe an irritated and inflamed bladder or kidneys. Pour one cup of boiling water over two teaspoons of fresh basil and birch leaves. Let it steep for about 10 minutes. Drink one cup three times a day between meals until the symptoms disappear.

You can add more basil to your diet in soups, Italian hoagies, stews, curries, pesto, and tea (turn to chapter 6 for some recipes).

Basil for reducing stress and anxiety

According to the *Journal of Ayurveda and Integrative Medicine*, holy basil has an antidepressant and anti-anxiety property comparable to diazepam and other antidepressant drugs. These studies showed that people who took 500 milligrams of holy basil extract each day felt less anxiety, stress, and depression; and these people became more social. Ayurvedic practitioners recommended drinking holy basil as tea using the leaves, and since it's caffeine free, its recommended to drink daily. The act of drinking tea is ritualistic and can be as calming as yoga. It fosters clear thought relaxation and a sense of wellbeing. Studies have shown that it can help people feel more social and less anxious.

Basil contains antibacterial properties

Researchers from the Medical University of Lodz in Poland tested the antibacterial activity of basil oil against strains of E. coli and other powerful bacteria that were gathered from sick patients with infections. The results showed that basil was effective in acting against the bacteria strains and helped to inhibit their growth. This has encouraged researchers to continue to study how basil and other antibacterial oils may help fight antibiotic resistant illnesses and infections.

Promotes cardiovascular health

Both as an antioxidant and anti-inflammatory food, basil can help the muscles that control blood pressure. Benefits of basil include the ability to help prevent dangerous platelet aggregation, clumping together of blood platelets that can form a clot within the arteries and cause cardiac arrest. Some of this is because of the vitamin K, magnesium, and beta-carotene. A study in *Oxidative Medicine and Cellular Longevity* concluded that rats fed basil daily for four weeks had reduced blood pressure. *The American Journal of Clinical Nutrition* concluded that diets that had magnesium had reduced blood pressure. The journal *Evidence-Based Complementary and Alternative Medicine* found that basil reduced the stress in 158 men and women.

Helps protect against diabetes and metabolic syndrome

When researchers from the Department of Home Science at Azad University of Agriculture and Technology in India investigated the effects of holy basil leaves on blood glucose and serum cholesterol levels in humans through double blind clinical trials, the results showed that basil caused significant improvements in blood glucose control and mild improvements in cholesterol. Some researchers think that holy basil may be able to help the body increase insulin production but more research as to be done to prove this theory.

# Sage

Sage is native to the northern Mediterranean coast. This widely cultivated herb is hardy north into Canada. The sage plant has gray-green edible leaves and flowers that can range in color from blue and purple to white or pink. There are more than nine hundred species of sage around the world. Sage has a long history of medicinal use for ailments ranging from mental disorders to gastrointestinal discomfort.

Benefits of sage

Sage can help protect the body's cells from damage caused by free radicals due to high antioxidant capacity. Free radicals often cause cells to die and can lead to impaired immunity and chronic disease. In laboratory studies, sage is active against several infection-causing bacteria. This fining lends some credence to the herb's age-old use in treating wounds. Modern physicians would not recommend bandaging with sage leaves. However, it is traditional treatment to use fresh leaves as garden first aid for minor wounds. Sage preservation may prevent food poisoning on your next picnic. Mix it generously into hamburger meat, tuna, pasta, and potato salad. As an antispasmodic, sage should theoretically calm the uterus. Some studies show that it does the opposite. The traditional role for sage is in menstruation promotion. Pregnant women should not take medicinal doses of sage. But some women may find it useful to bring on their periods. Some women have used sage to improve the symptoms of menopause, including hot flashes. Sage cools the body and reduces perspiration. A 2011 study by S. Bommer, P Klein and A. Suter showed a 50 percent improvement after four weeks and a 64 percent improvement after eight weeks. The antibacterial actions of sage work best in the mouth and throat. Many have used it for sore and swollen gums in gingivitis. In the 2015 *Iranian Journal of Microbiology*, a sage mouthwash was shown to significantly reduce the amounts of Streptococcus mutans in dental plaque. The Oregon Health and Science University published a study in 2017 using sage for Alzheimer's disease. Over a four-month period, patients taking 60 drops of Salvia liquid a day had significantly better cognitive function as measured by the Alzheimer's disease assessment scale than patients taking a placebo. The British did a study on sage and young people for memory. In the journal *Pharmacological Biochemical Behavior*, they concluded that a 50-microliter dose of sage improved word recall. Sage can aid in lowering cholesterol and blood glucose. There is a 2013 study published in *Complementary Therapies in Medicine* that reported patients given sage had a lower fasting glucose and lower triglyceride and LDL but higher HDL after three months of treatment.

How sage is used

There are several ways to use sage. You can drink it in teas or put it in mulled wine or cider. With tea, you may want to add honey to sweeten the bitter taste. You can eat it by adding it to roasted vegetables, put it in stuffing or dressings with poultry, add it to pesto, put it in baked goods, or add it to salad dressings. You can put it in steams for your sinuses. You can add it to butter for basting fish or with pasta or rice. You can use it to purify rooms for the sick room or other rooms to invigorate the energy. Or you can use it as a spritzer along with rosemary to stimulate your face or scalp. You can also put some in your bath water to help you fight off infections, stimulate circulation, and relieve pain.

Smudging

Some cultures use smudging to purify rooms from sickness or even bad luck. It turns out that this may have some scientific basis. In the 2006 *Journal of Ethnopharmacology*, in an article titled "Medicinal Sage Smoke May Have a Broad Range of Therapeutic Applications and Benefits." The article concluded that "the advantages of smoke-based remedies are rapid delivery to the brain, more efficient absorption by the body and lower costs of production." In the same journal a year later in an article called, "Medicinal Smokes," concluded that the smoke did indeed kill 94 percent of bacteria in the air. Sage smoke may also improve your mood and lift your spirits. In 2016, the University of Mississippi did a study of white sage had compounds that relieved mood, reduced stress, and even alleviated pain. They found it could even improve sleep and relieve anxiety. Don't inhale the smoke directly and leave a window open while smudging. Perhaps in our world of overusing antibiotic sprays and cleaning products, it may be time to change to essential oils. In addition, smudging adds negative ions to the air that work on par with antidepressants for mood disorders and improve physical performance. This is according to *Research in Psychology and Behavioral Sciences*, 2013.

## Sage Tea

*Sage tea may be one of the easiest ways to get the benefits of sage. It will help you detoxify by stimulating your kidney and liver.*

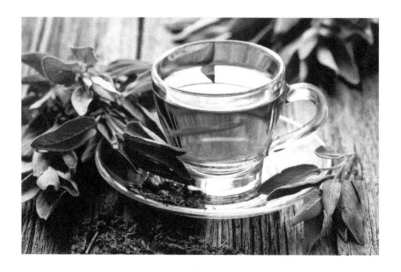

2 teaspoons of fresh sage leaves or 1 teaspoon of dried sage leaves
1 cup of filtered water
Honey, lemon, or orange slices for taste

Bring the water to a high simmer, and then remove the pot from the heat. Add the sage leaves in the water to steep for 5 to 8 minutes. Strain the mixture to remove the leaves. Add the honey, orange, or lemon to improve the taste.

# Onion

Onion: the super plant

Which plant is most often depicted in Egyptian tombs paintings? Which plant did the Greeks and Romans have a love-hate relationship with, praising its healing properties but damning its rank odor? Which plant did Alexander the Great feed to his troops to give them strength before battle? The answer is the onion!

Most researchers agree the onion has been cultivated for five thousand years or more. Since onions grew wild in various regions, they were probably consumed for thousands of years and domesticated simultaneously all over the world. Onions may be one of the earliest cultivated crops because they were less perishable than other foods of that time. They were transportable. They were easy to grow and could be grown in a variety of soils and climates.

In Egypt, onions were considered an object of worship. The onion symbolized eternity to the Egyptians who buried onions, along with their pharaohs. The Egyptian saw eternal life in the anatomy of onion because of its circles within a circle structure. Paintings of onions appear on the inner walls of pyramids and the tombs of both the Old Kingdom and the New Kingdom.

Varieties of onion

In India, as early as the sixth century BC, the famous medical treatise, Charaka-Sanhita celebrates the onion as medicine, a diuretic, food for digestion, the heart, the eyes, and the joints. Onions were eaten by Israelites in the Bible. Ancient Romans ate onions regularly and brought them on their journeys of conquest in England and much of Central Europe.

Components of onion

According to the US Food and Drug Administration, a medium onion contains the following:

-   45 calories and no fat and no cholesterol
-   11 grams of carbohydrates (4 percent of the RDI)
-   Dietary fiber: 3 grams
-   Sugar: 9 grams
-   Iron (4 percent of the RDI)
-   Potassium 190 mg (5 percent of the RDI)
-   Protein (1 percent of the RDI)
-   Vitamin C (20 percent of the RDI)
-   Calcium (4 percent of the RDI)

Health benefits of onions

*Improves your skin.* Onion is one of the richest sources of quercetin, the most powerful antioxidant that can keep your skin wrinkle-free. Vitamins and sulfur on the hand protect your skin and keep it soft and supple. The anti-aging qualities of onions can be attributed to the presence of sulfur-rich phytochemicals. Massaging your skin with fresh onion juice helps increase blood circulation and improves the overall appearance of skin.

*Helps you to take care of acne and other skin problems.* Onions can be used in the treatment of acne and pimples. For this purpose, you can mix a tablespoon of onion juice or extract with a tablespoon of olive oil and apply it to your face. Leave on for twenty minutes, then wash it off. Onions are great for dark spots and skin pigmentation. You can prepare an onion face mask by mixing equal quantities of onion juice and fresh yogurt. You can also add a few drops of any essential oil for a pleasant aroma. Massage your face with this mixture, using gentle circular movements for ten to fifteen minutes. This should be done daily for the best result.

*Helps you cure coughs.* Onions are great for coughs. Honey mixed with onion juice was widely used as a healing tonic during the

Great Depression, when few folks could afford drugstore remedies. Honey or sugar is used in this tonic to draw the juice from the onion and simulate saliva flow. This helps you clear your throat and reduce inflammation. You can slice an onion into rings and place in a deep bowl and cover with honey. Let this sit for ten to twelve hours. Then strain out the onion, and take one tablespoon of the resulting syrup four or five times a day. You can also chop the onions finely with about half as much honey and half cup of sugar. Again, strain and use four to five times a day.

*Contains healthful chemicals.* Red onions, in particular, contain antioxidants, which give them their distinct purple color. These healthful chemicals are more concentrated on the outer flesh of the onions. Over-peeling onions could lead to losses of about 20 percent of quercetin and 75 percent of anthocyanins. The sulfur compounds are responsible for the smell of onions. They make your eyes water when you cut the onion. These sulfur compounds also can protect you against cancer, inhibit the growth of microorganisms, and prevent the formation of blood clots. Your colon cancer risk can be further reduced by adding turmeric to your diet.

*Contains vitamins.* Onions contain vitamin C, folic acid, vitamin B6, and potassium. The vitamins are mostly lost in cooking, but you are sure to get their benefits if you eat them raw.

*Improves oral health.* Raw onions may make our breath stink, but they can actually improve our oral health. Simply chewing a raw onion can strengthen teeth and eliminate bacteria that can lead to tooth decay. Two of three minutes of chewing on an onion can kill most germs in the mouth.

*Helps you with blood sugar.* Onions can regulate blood sugar. According to a March 6, 2015, *Science News*, a study of using onion extract was used on diabetic rats. "Two doses of onion extract, 400 and 600 mg/kg/day, strongly reduced fasting blood sugar levels in diabetic rats by 50 percent and 35 percent, respectively, compared with baseline levels at the start of the study before the rodents received onion extract," Ojieh reported.

*Can be used as treatment for alopecia areata. The Journal of Dermatology,* July 22, 2014, discussed onions as a topical treatment for alopecia areata. In patchy alopecia, 86.9 percent of patients had hair re-growth after applying onion juice for six weeks. To make the juice, peel the onions, and cut them into quarters. Blend in a juicer and add a little water. Then filter the juice with a muslin cloth. Massage into scalp and let sit for one hour. Then rinse it off with a mild shampoo with nice fragrance.

## Summary

Herbal remedies have been used for five thousand years. The herbs mentioned here are not the only ones, but they are among the best ones. Cayenne pepper, garlic, aloe vera, echinacea, ginger, basil, sage, and onion are some of the best plant medicine on the planet. They come from all over the world, including India, China, Egypt, Greece, Rome, and Native Americans. These cures existed before modern medicine. Some are now being reexamined under the eyes of modern science and found useful.

However, herbs are not regulated like medicines and amounts not always precise. Some places sell herbs that are improperly labeled or may not be the exact herb that the label claims it to be. Always consult a medical professional before using herbs in place of a medicine or if you are using it for healing of an ailment.

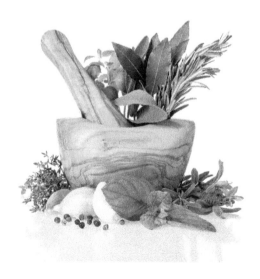

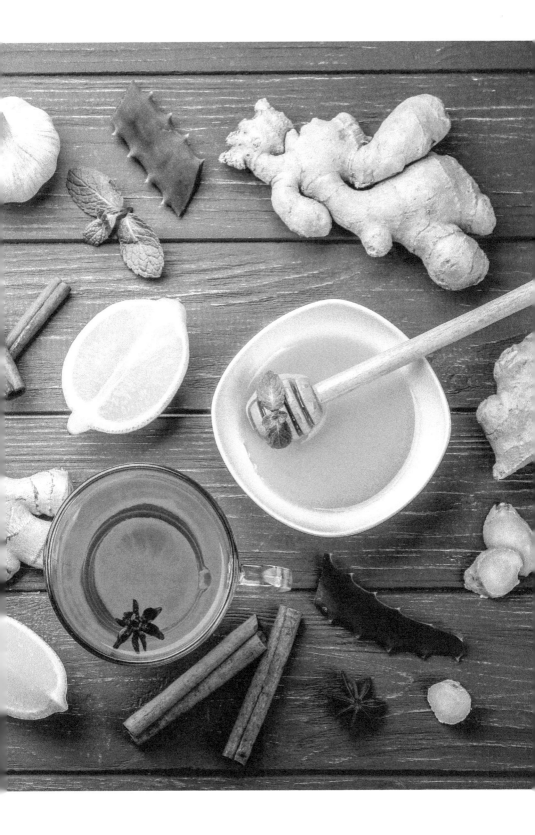

# Chapter 8

# The Power of Your Mind

Our mind is an incredibly powerful tool. We only use a small portion of it. Researchers have proven that our mental state has a direct impact on our body.

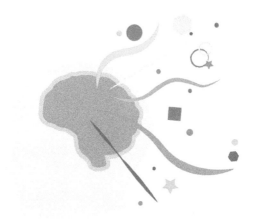

## Mind/Body Medicine

Physical and mental stimulation activities

If you are stressed or worried, you have an increased chance of getting sick. The mind is extremely powerful; and when used correctly, it will help you get back on track, discover what you want and why, and can help you start discovering wonderful opportunities in your life. How is that possible? Your subconscious mind is a second, hidden mind that exists within you. It interprets and acts upon the predominating thoughts that reside within your conscious mind, and its goal is to attract circumstances and situations that match the images you have within. Your thoughts and beliefs are like seeds in the garden, and the content of your thoughts will have an effect on your life. We create what we think, and what we think sends out a vibration that attracts similar thoughts and people who share similar thoughts. Beliefs have powerful vibrations that will quickly manifest results in your life. If you constantly say that you are unsure or do not know what to do, you will create more confusion, and you will attract situations that will confuse you even more. Stop this never-ending cycle of confusion and begin thinking about what you want. Begin creating the right vibrations and the right energy to attract the opportunities, people, and situations to help you achieve your goals.

Stronger than circumstances

Does this describe your life:

- Do you jump out of bed every morning, energized and thrilled about starting the day?
- Do you enjoy vibrant health, deep love, time, freedom, and financial abundance?
- Is your life fulfilling, expanded, and purposeful?
- Does your life inspire you and bring you joy?
- Do you have the freedom and confidence of knowing you can accomplish anything you want?

Your best life is within your reach, but what is keeping you from it? The problem is that you have done nothing differently. The ideas, techniques, and strategies are all there in your head; but you are not using them to make the changes you thought you would make. That's because your paradigm is working full-time to prevent you from making changes. If you don't know how to spot its "tricks," you might fall for them without even knowing it.

Whenever you start to move toward the life you desire, your subconscious mind (ego) comes at you with the three following dream-busting paradigms.

1. Distraction

- You have a meeting first thing on Monday morning, so you should think about that right now.
- You will be more creative if you get your laundry done and your desk cleared off first.
- You will be able to build your dream better if you are not hungry. How about some lunch now?
- You have not checked your phone in ten minutes. Maybe there is an important message you should read first?

Your paradigm won't bust through the doors of your mind yelling, "Stop taking steps toward your dream!" It just does what it does best. It distracts you!

2. Discussion

If your paradigm cannot distract you, it will come at you with a different tactic. It's going to dissuade you with the common catch-phrase, "I actually don't want to..."

Assume you wanted to be promoted at your job. You thought about setting up a meeting with your boss to discuss future opportunities, but before you could make the call, you found yourself saying, "I'm busy enough as it is. I do not want the added stress. The raise in pay won't make that much of a difference. You know, maybe I don't want the promotion." The goal you set for yourself will be forgotten, and you will never accomplish it.

The challenge is that your paradigm knows everything about you. It remembers all the times when you didn't do what you said you were going to do. It has access to the whole filing cabinet of failed attempts, forgotten dreams, and unrealized goals.

3.   DEFCON 1

If your paradigm can't stop you through distraction or dissuasion, it's going to try one last tactic. It's going to trigger "DEFCON 1," or your fight or flight reflex, which is difficult to ignore. You are going to feel an uncontrollable or irrational fear, which has the capacity to stop you dead in your tracks when you are building your dream.

DEFCON 1 is a United States military term that stands for "defense readiness condition," and number 1 is the highest state of alertness in times of national security threats. When you are in this state, you might begin to feel flushed, jittery, or panicked, and not know why.

See if you can relate to any of these circumstances:

You pick up the phone to make an important call. Suddenly, you feel butterflies in your stomach, and you either stare at the phone unable to dial or you hang up before anyone answers. You have gotten up every morning to exercise, but on day 8, you hit the wall. You are completely drained of energy and feel angry that you don't see any results yet. When DEFCON 1 happens, you may be tempted to rush back to the familiar because in the moment, your feelings are alarming. The familiar may be your daily routine, a "safe" job, an "okay" relationship, or the comforts of your current home.

These tactics are very convincing, and they can crush your dreams if you are not alert. Fortunately, there are ways you can overcome the insidious forces of your paradigm and quickly and easily begin to live your dream. The truth is, everyone has a paradigm because it is a part of human nature. Most people stay stagnant because after many failed attempts to overcome their paradigm, they have given up on living their dream.

Here are some effective tools to help rewire your mind for success:

- "Your past is gone. Your mistakes are behind you. Focus on your gorgeous, love-filled future. The only thing you are responsible for now is taking each step with intention. Rebuild your life. Make it gold" (Cara Alwill Leybe).
- Note your thoughts and feelings. If you have any of the following thoughts, know that your paradigm is operating its agenda:

  - *It has always been like this…*
  - *It's so hard to…*
  - *I've never been able to…*
  - *I always do this…*
  - *I can't…*

These thoughts are called "systems," and they reinforce your paradigm. When you notice these thoughts, first acknowledge them without judgment. Now, you can start to repattern them.

My teacher, Mary Morrissey, recommended repatterning my thoughts by using three magic words, *up until now*, at the end. For example, "I cannot do…up until now." "I have never been able to… up until now."

In order to make changes in your life, you must change the way you use your mind. You cannot think both negative and positive thoughts at the same time. As humans, we are creatures of habit, and so are our minds. Most people think that changing external conditions by working the same way will help. But first you have to change the internal. Train your conscious mind to think thoughts of success, happiness, health, and prosperity. Learn to weed out negativity, such as fear and worry. Keep your conscious mind busy with the expectation of the best. Keep your thoughts based upon what you want in your life.

Principles of mind/body medicine

Studies suggest that human beings are not biological robots, controlled entirely by genes and the conditioning of life experiences. Eastern traditions (Ayurveda, qigong, yoga) have for centuries believed that consciousness plays an essential role in governing physical and psychological health. Why? Each person is unique. No two people are alike, so even if they have the same disease, the path to recovery may be different. They come from different parents, were raised by different traditions, and their minds and bodies are different.

Taking self-responsibility for healing

The body has a natural biological tendency to move toward health and balance. Those who have positive thoughts will get better. This healing power helps everyone. Biofeedback research, for example, has shown that individuals can learn to control brainwave activity, affect cardiovascular and respiratory functioning, and reduce skin temperature. Using mind power is a new healing philosophy. Relaxation, stress reduction, guided imagery, and behavioral change are the best things you can do for yourself.

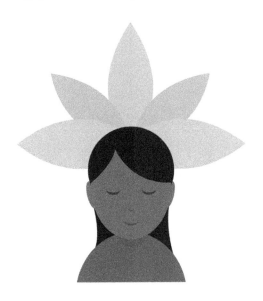

# Yoga

Yoga dates back to approximately 1500 BC in the Vedic period. Composed in Vedic Sanskrit, the Vedas are the oldest writings of Hinduism and Sanskrit literature. The Vedas actually refers to a yoke, as in the yoke over animals—and at times a chariot in the midst of battle.

Yoga is the union of mind, spirit, and body. Yoga comes from the Hindu philosophy used to attain spiritual insight and harmony. It is a fantastic remedy for overcoming the problems that modern humans face in daily life. Yoga helps to enhance the autoimmune system, and it increases the vital energy in the body system.

How often do we find that we are unable to perform our activities properly because of confusion and conflicts in our mind weighing heavily down upon us? Stress is the number one culprit affecting all the parts of our physical, endocrinal, and emotional systems. With the help of yoga, these things can be corrected. Yoga can help you create a sense of calmness and well-being. Yoga exercise helps you improve your circulation. Your organs and veins need to be exercised to function properly.

Yoga can help stimulate your immune system and keep you disease-free!

General benefits of yoga

1.  Physical

    -   Creates a flexible and strong body
    -   Helps to maintain a balanced metabolism

2.  Mental

    -   Helps you relax and handle stressful situations easily
    -   Encourages positive thoughts and self-acceptance

3. Spiritual

- Builds awareness of your body
- Promotes an inter-dependence between mind, body, and spirit

Five years ago, I started my first yoga class. I spent most of the time watching everyone else, as I had no idea how it worked or what the poses were. Some of the postures even caused discomfort. Time is the best doctor. I practiced more and learned more, and I made progress. I have spent the last two years practicing yoga at my home, and it is now a part of my life. It has made me confident inside and out so that I can face people without worry. I have also experienced increased muscle tone, strength, and flexibility.

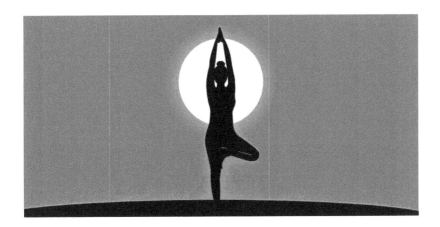

These are twelve yoga poses that I suggest for beginners:

1. Downward-facing dog/*adho mukha svanasana*

    • Start on your hands and knees with hands stacked under your shoulders and knees under your hips.
    • Spread your hands wide, and press your index finger and thumb into your mat. Lift your tailbone and press your butt up and back, drawing your

hips toward the ceiling. Straighten your legs as best as you can and press your heels gently toward the floor.

- Your head should be between your arms, facing your knees, and your back should be flat.
- Hold for five to ten breaths.

2. Mountain pose/*tadasana*

- Stand with toes and heels slightly apart.
- Spread your toes, and place your weight evenly between both feet. Engage your core and tuck your hips under a bit so your tailbone is pointing down toward the floor. Relax your shoulders and roll them back and down.
- Inhale and reach your arms overhead while pressing into your feet. You may also put your hands into a prayer position in front of your chest or rest them by your sides. All of these are commonly used variations.
- Take long, slow, deep breaths, in and out of your nose.
- Hold for three to five breaths.

3. Crescent lunge/*utthita ashwa sanchalansana*

- Take a big step forward with your left foot to start in a staggered stance, with your feet almost mat-length apart.
- Bend your front knee and keep your back leg straight and heel lifted off the floor. Try to bend your front leg so that your thigh is parallel to the floor. Square your hips toward the front.

4. Warrior II/*virabhadrasana II*

- Take a big step forward with your left foot to start in a staggered stance, with your feet almost mat-length.
- Extend your arms so that they are parallel to the floor.
- Bend your left knee so that it's at or near a ninety-degree angle, your thigh parallel to the floor, while keeping the right leg straight.
- Point your left toes forward and turn your right foot out to the right so that it's perpendicular to your left foot. Your left heel should be in line with the arch of your right foot.
- At the same time, twist your torso to the right so that your left hip is facing toward the front of the room and your right hip is facing toward the back. Your left arm and your head should both be pointing forward and your right arm should be pointing back.
- Hold for one to five breaths.

5. Triangle/*trikonasana*

- Start in warrior II position.
- Straighten your front leg. Then reach forward with your left hand toward the ground. Tilt your torso forward, and rotate it open to the right side.
- Rotate your arms to six and twelve o'clock. Rest your left hand on your shin or the floor if you can. Extend your top arm fingers toward the ceiling.
- Hold for five to ten breaths, then switch sides.

6. Plank pose/*kumbhakasana*

- Start on all fours, with your knees under your hips and your hands flat on the floor directly underneath your shoulders.
- Lift your knees off the floor and extend your legs out behind you. You should now be on your toes and your hands, with your body forming one long line.
- Keep your palms flat on the floor, hands shoulder-width apart, shoulders stacked directly above your wrists, and core engaged. Keep your neck and spine in neutral position by looking down at the top of your mat.
- Hold this position for three to five breaths.

7. Low plank/*chaturanga dandasana*

- Start in plank pose with your palms flat on the floor, hands shoulder-width apart, shoulders stacked directly above your wrists, legs extended, and core engaged.
- Slowly lower down to a low plank by bending your elbows, keeping them tucked in close to the side of your body, until they form ninety-degree angles. Hold for one breath.

8. Upward-facing dog/*urdhva mukha svansana*

- From low plank/chaturanga, drop your hips down to the floor, and flip your toes over so the tops of your feet touch the floor.
- Tighten your core and straighten your arms to push your chest up. Pull your shoulders back, squeeze your shoulder blades, and tilt your head toward the ceiling to open up your chest.

9. Tree/*vrksasana*

- Start in mountain pose with your toes together and heels slightly apart.
- Bring your right foot to the inner thigh of your left leg. Squeeze your foot and inner thigh together. The knee of your right leg should be turned out and your right thigh facing down toward the ground at a forty-five-degree angle.
- Once you have found your balance, lift your hands to prayer position in front of your chest.
- Keep your gaze focused on a fixed point in front of you to help keep you balanced.
- Hold for five to ten breaths, then switch sides.

10. Dancers pose/*natarajasana*

- Stand tall with your feet together.
- Bend your left knee, and bring your left foot toward your glutes. Grab onto the inner arch of your left foot with your left hand, and slowly lift your foot toward the ceiling. At the same time, reach your right arm forward and up toward the ceiling.
- Actively press down into the floor with entire right foot as you start to open your chest and pull your lifted leg up. Keep your chest lifted.
- Hold on one side for five to ten breaths, and then switch sides.

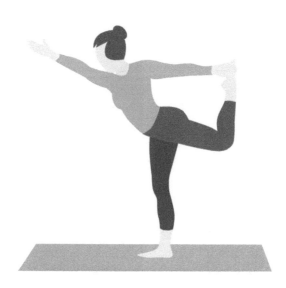

11.  Half pigeon pose/*ardha kapotasana*

    •   From downward-facing dog, extend your left leg high, and then bring your leg underneath your body, and place it in front of you (with your shin parallel to the top of your mat).
    •   Extend your right leg straight behind you. Rest the top of your foot on the floor.
    •   Keep your left foot flexed. Try to keep your right hip as close to the mat as you can. If it lifts off the floor, bring your left foot in a little closer to your body.
    •   Stay upright for three breaths. Then fold over, and rest your head on the ground for five to ten breaths.
    •   Repeat on the other leg.

12.  Seated forward fold/*paschimottanasana*

    •   Sit on the floor with your legs extended in front of you. Flex your feet. Sit up tall with a straight back.

- Bending from your hips and keeping your back flat, fold your upper body over your lower body.
- If you are able to, grab onto the outside of each foot, or your ankles or shins. Release your neck and let your head hang heavy.
- Hold for five to ten breaths.

Yoga is done bare foot on a yoga mat. Even the most basic yoga stretches require clothes that can stretch or move, so wear the most comfortable outfit that allows you to move easily. If you attend a class at a studio, they will provide everything you need. However, if you are doing a class online, you will need a yoga mat. Yoga is accessible for everyone—no matter what you look like, how old you are, how you dress, or what religion you practice. Try it! It's fun and healthy!

*Yoga and fitness go hand in hand.*

## Fitness

Our thoughts, feelings, beliefs, and obsessions drive our actions and behaviors. True fitness is not just physical. Training yourself will get your body into dramatically better shape, but the physical changes will be just a small part of a much bigger transformation. Total fitness is about getting healthier and stronger throughout your life.

Total fitness will keep your mind and spirit strong and healthy. It will give you self-respect, self-acceptance, and self-appreciation that comes from knowing you can achieve the goals you set for yourself. This means that you should get every part of your mind and body in shape so that you can start to live the life you want and deserve. We are creatures of habit, programmed according to our past conditioning. We eat dinner every night whether we are hungry or not, and we have dessert whether we are full or not because that is what we have always done. Even though we know better, we continue to treat our disappointments with junk food parties in front of the TV. We often use our moods and disappointments to stay stuck in the same place. We often tell ourselves that things will always be the same or that we are not deserving of a better life. Nobody can keep you from believing that you deserve a better life. There is no surgery for changing our minds, our beliefs, or what we see when we look at ourselves with our inner eye. Fitness for your body and mind is no more difficult than things you have done in the past. The mind does not follow the body. The body follows the mind. Your thoughts and beliefs create and support your behaviors, not the other way around. Your body needs repetition and conditioning to change, and your mind does too. I recommend that my clients meditate, repeat mantras, chant, read affirmations, or pray for ten minutes two times per day. These practices have been utilized and followed for thousands and thousands of years—because they work. Your health and your happiness depend on the fitness of your body, mind, and spirit. You need to create your fitness.

Walking for fitness: is it for you?

Millions of Americans can easily include walking in their fitness programs because walking requires only two things, properly fitting athletic shoes and somewhere to walk (a scenic path, or perhaps a shopping mall, indoor track, or treadmill in case of a bad weather).

Getting started walking

- You can start a fitness walking program in fitness workshops.
- Find a friend who will accompany you on your fitness walks.
- Join a local fitness walking group.
- Make walking an everyday habit like brushing your teeth or combing your hair.
- Schedule walks into your day.
- Set both short and long-term goals.
- Reward yourself for reaching a short-term goal.
- Treat yourself to a massage or a new shirt.
- Be your own coach.

The right shoes

- Purchase athletic shoes from a reputable business that specializes in athletic footwear.
- Look for a high and wide-toe box.
- Look for a walking shoe with a cushioned, flexible sole and a top/upper that lets the foot breathe or allows air to circulate around the foot and moisture to escape.
- Be sure the shoe has good traction and is capable of absorbing shock.
- Be sure to try on shoes in the store. Wear the socks you will walk in, and walk around a while before you decide.

Choosing appropriate socks is important. Wear athletic socks that are adequately cushioned and have effective "wicking" properties (they draw the perspiration away from your foot). Choosing appropriate clothing for walking depends on the weather. Dress in layers suitable to the weather, so you can add or remove clothing if the weather changes during your workout or as your body temperature changes with the intensity of your workout. Reflective clothing is always a good idea, even in the daytime.

Walking basics

When you are walking the way your foot strikes, the ground is important if you want to get the best workout possible and avoid injury. When your foot strikes the ground, roll over your heel instead of hitting the ground with it. Your posture while you walk is also very important. Keep your chin level with the ground. Walk tall, and drop your shoulders naturally.

How long should you walk?

First, warm up by walking at your usual walking place for five to seven minutes. After you have warmed up, note what time it is. This is the beginning of your exercise period. Walk about twenty minutes, then increase intensity. Keep at this until you feel uncomfortable or breathless. After you feel uncomfortable, walk slowly for five to seven minutes.

The benefits of walking:

- Promotes and maintains weight loss
- Promotes cardiovascular health
- Promotes ideal posture
- Improve flexibility
- Boosts mood and energy
- Reduces risk of osteoporosis

Keep walking during your recovery period. Listen to your body, and see how it feels. Do not give in to your old ways. Honor yourself, and you will get the best results for your health. One of the best things about walking is that you can do it anywhere—you can hike in hills, hit the neighborhood, go to a gym, a park, a school track, or do laps around the mall.

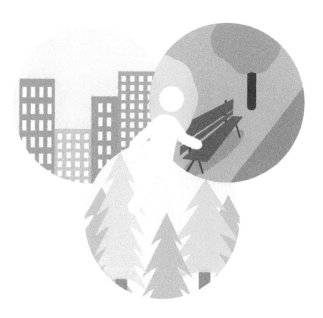

# Hydrotherapy

Hydrotherapy is the use of water, ice, steam, and hot or cold temperatures to maintain and restore health. Hydrotherapy is effective for treating a wide range of conditions and can easily be used in the home as part of a self-care program. Hydrotherapy, also called water therapy or physiotherapy, is a form of alternative medicine involving the use of water to revitalize, restore, and maintain health. In most types of hydrotherapy treatments, water is either directly applied to the skin, or the body is immerged into hot or cold water. Specifically, naturopathic hydrotherapy uses alternating applications of hot and cold water to increase blood flow and improve circulation.

Hydrotherapy's main rule of healing is rooted in the role that it serves in the body. Blood runs to every cell, tissue, and organ in the human system and provides oxygen and nutrients to sustain the cells of the body. The blood is the medium for detoxification, taking harmful toxins from cells and excreting them out through the urine. With application of hot and cold water treatments, the circulation of the blood and the proliferation of blood components are improved, thus making the body more efficient in restoring needed nutrients and oxygen to areas of the body that needs healing. Throughout history, hydrotherapy has been universally adopted in many diverse cultures. From the Old Testament to the ancient Greeks, water has been used as a therapeutic agent and has been thought to have healing power. In the early 1920s, President D. Roosevelt embraced the ancient practice as the main form of therapy to treat his polio and regained worldwide attention to hydrotherapy. Today, hydrotherapy is used as an alternative medicine for the treatment of arthritis, depression, stress, sleep disorders, and for joint, muscle, and nerve problems.

How hydrotherapy works

We have some natural healing waters that spring from the earth. The balances of minerals in seawater are similar to that of human blood. The water from natural springs carries concentrated levels of sodium, calcium, magnesium, bicarbonate, and sulfur. Bicarbonate spring water can aid cuts, burns, hardening of the skin, digestive problems, and allergies. Sulfur has been known to help arthritis, rheumatism, chronic poisoning, diabetes, skin disease, and urinary disease. Hydrotherapy techniques are used in spas and therapy centers around the world, according to Dr. Burton Goldberg (from *Alternative Medicine*).

Many treatments of hydrotherapy can be used at home.

Ice and contrast

Effective therapies for trauma relief. Any injury, like sprains, strains, inflammation, or tendinitis, can be helped by the application of cold. Apply ice as often as twenty minutes every hour for the first twenty-four to thirty-six hours after the trauma.

Trauma or chronic conditions also respond well to contrast therapy. Alternating hot and cold increases circulation to bring vital nutrients to the area and move waste products out. Simply apply alternating hot and cold packs to the affected area, beginning with hot for three minutes, then cold for thirty to sixty seconds. Repeat three times in one sitting. Always finish with cold water, treating one to three times per day.

Sitz baths

A traditional European folk remedy in which the pelvis is immersed in hot or cold water, a hot sitz bath is helpful for problems involving the pelvic region, including uterine cramps and hemorrhoids.

Foot and hand baths

Excellent for drawing blood away from inflamed parts of the body or drawing congestion away from an organ, they can help relieve insomnia, sore throats, colds, menstrual cramps, feet and leg cramps, and pain from gout. Alternating hot and cold foot baths has a good effect on the nerve and reflex points of the feet. These baths help relieve toothaches, neuralgia, headaches, ankle swelling, foot infections, and abdominal congestion.

Fill two tubs, one with hot water, the other with cold water. Place your feet and ankles in the hot water for three minutes, then plunge your feet into the cold water for twenty to thirty seconds. Repeat three times, ending with cold water, then thoroughly dry your feet. You may do this several times per day, as needed. Hands also contain many reflex points that affect the entire body. A cold hand bath can stop a nosebleed and relieve sunstroke. A hot hand bath can relieve cramps in the hands from overuse in athletics, writing, or sewing, and also alleviate asthma attacks.

Healing baths

A number of herbs, essential oils, and minerals may be added to a bath to enhance its therapeutic effects. A few drops of various essential oils may also be added to the bath or rubbed directly onto the skin after a shower. According to Dr. Chaitow, they influence blood pressure and stimulate nerve and digestive functioning.

Here are a few of the more common herbs used in hydrotherapy, available at most natural food stores:

- Ginger relaxes sore muscles, improves circulation, and tones the skin.
- Sage stimulates the sweat glands.
- Cedar wood promotes elimination through mucous membranes and acts as an antiseptic.
- Rose stimulates liver and stomach function and acts as an antidepressant.
- Tea tree enhances skin function and can be used as an antifungal and an antibiotic.
- Apple cider vinegar detoxifies, combats fatigue, relieves poison ivy, and restores the skin's natural acid covering. Add one cup to your bath.

- Baking soda relieves skin irritation and itching, and acts as a mild antiseptic. Add one pound to hot bath.
- Cornstarch helps reduce itchiness from poison ivy, poison oak, and eczema. Add one cup to one pond of cornstarch to the bath.
- Oatmeal soothes and restores the skin and is especially good for itchiness, hives, and sunburn. Put one cup of uncooked oatmeal in a blender, finely blend it, and add it to warm bath.

Heating compresses

A heating compress is a cold application that is left in place for a long period of time. It is heated by the body and then becomes a hot application. The heating compress requires an active response from the body and therefore stimulates increased metabolic and healing activity in its vicinity. Because it encourages blood flow into an area, it can be used to reduce congestion in another area. To bring blood into an area makes it useful for treating chronic joint pain or chronic bronchitis. It can be used in treating acute and chronic sore throat, tonsillitis, and ear infection.

Cold water treating

One of the "most important preventive water treatments," says Dr. Dian Dincin Buchman. After a shower or bath, immerse your feet in cold water and walk in place for five seconds to five minutes. Afterward, rub your feet vigorously with a towel, especially the soles. Dr. Buchman believes that by building tolerance to cold, it is possible to develop resistance to infectious disease. She recommends this practice be a part of the daily self-care routine for everyone, young or old.

Steam

An excellent cleanser and deep moisture treatment for the skin. It helps break up congestion from colds and the flu. To create a simple home vaporizer, boil water in a clean kettle or pan. Add a few drops of eucalyptus or wintergreen oil or one to two tablespoons of mint leaves to the water. Lean over the steaming pot, holding a towel or sheet over your head like a tent. Be careful not to get too close to the boiling water. Breathe slowly and deeply, inhaling the vapors to warm and soothe the respiratory tract.

Creating a heating compress

Materials needed: one pair light cotton socks, one pair heavy wool or acrylic socks, or a lightweight cotton fabric cut in width and length to wrap around the area to be treated (joint, neck, etc.). You will also need a wool cloth, cotton t-shirt, or wool sweater to cover the body.

Procedure: This wet sock treatment is especially useful in treating children with upper respiratory infections. Before bedtime, wring a pair of cotton socks in ice water, pull over feet, and cover with wool socks. Leave in place overnight. By morning, the socks should be warm and dry.

One can use a chest pack on the chest and cover yourself with a wool sweater. Leave in place overnight.

Knee, ankle, and throat conditions may be treated by wrapping the area with a cotton cloth wrung from cold water and covered with wool. Leave for several hours.

Dr. Lewis says,

> In Europe, hydrotherapy is commonly found in health clinics, both as a primary and an adjunctive treatment modality. In the United States, there is also a definite resurgence of interest in hydrotherapy, which I feel is due to the growing dissatisfaction people have with the overuse of medication. People are looking for other alternatives."

# Crystal Healing

Since ancient times, crystals have been used for their powerful energetic healing properties. Crystals are naturally occurring solids made from minerals; and they come in all shapes, sizes, and colors. Crystals can help heal deep-seated issues, bringing forth good health and greater happiness. Each crystal has its own unique healing properties. Some are best suited for abundance and prosperity while others are better for love, relationships, and harmony. There are even crystals for protection and shielding. Crystals provide a gentle, non-invasive form of healing that cooperates with your body's inner healer (a repair mechanism that brings your body back into balance). While crystals work quickly for minor ailments, such as headache, other conditions can take longer to heal. The habits of a lifetime and the ingrained attitudes that can underlie a disease, for instance, will not change overnight. With persistence, crystals can transmute these to bring about a lasting improvement in your condition. Crystal healing is most effective in helping you to uncover the psychosomatic causes of disease. Psychosomatic means that your emotions and mental attitudes are affecting your physical body and causing disease, and this is a situation which crystals can improve. The mind is closely involved in crystal healing. Belief in them speeds up the process, but you do not have to believe—merely to keep an open mind.

The Tibetans, like many ancient peoples, have used crystals for thousands of years and believe closed-mindedness is one of the major causes of disease. They also believe that the body has natural tendency toward wellness, that if you listen to your body, you instinctively know what is good for you. Crystal healing is an alternative medical technique in which crystals and other stones are used to cure ailments and protect against disease.

How does crystal healing work?

- Clearing: Crystals have the ability to absorb and remove certain types of energy from your body. Like a magnet can pick up little pieces of metal shavings, a healing crystal can absorb negative energy from your body.

- Energizing: Healing crystals and stones can also push energy into your body, mind, or spirit through inducing resonant frequencies. This is similar to the way electricity works by conducting and transferring energy into an object. Crystal healing is painless and not dangerous.
- Balancing: When you are under stress or are ill, your energy is out of balance. Healing crystals can be used to balance out areas of energetic disharmony.

Using the crystals

*Gem elixirs.* As crystals work by vibration and resonance, the energy can be easily transferred into water where it is stored until required.

How to make gem elixir:

- Cleanse your crystals before use.
- Place the crystal in a clean glass bowl, and cover them with pure spring water.
- Cover the bowl and place in the sun for six and a half hours.
- Remove the crystal.
- Keep elixir in the clean glass bottle and cap with an airtight stopper. Sip the elixir, use it in the bath, or put it in a bottle of water, and spray around your home or workplace.

Crystals for clearing and protection

Crystal vibrations are excellent for counteracting negative energy of all kinds: they stabilize excess energy and absorb toxicity, thus creating harmony within your home, workplace, or external surroundings.

- Smoky quartz

A smoky quartz crystal can be programmed and placed in your car to keep it and you safe at all times. Simply hold the crystal in your hands for a few moments, visualizing it surrounded by light and ask that it will afford protection to you, your passengers, and your car.

- Amethyst

Amethyst is one of the great protector stones. It brings a high spiritual vibration into your home, guarding against psychic attack and ill-wishing, blocks stress, and removes environmental pollution.

- Bloodstone

Bloodstone usually works on the physical body, but it also has the ability to block out undesirable influences. Place a bloodstone at each corner of your house to keep yourself safe.

- Orange carnelian

Orange carnelian kept close to the door attracts an abundance of good things to your home.

- Smoky quartz

Smoky quartz will mop up the negativity and replace it with brighter vibes.

- Sodalite

Sodalite absorbs the emanations of high-frequency communication, antennas, microwaves, and computers.

Crystals at work

- Blue lace agate quickly restores peace and harmony if there is discord within your working environment.

- Green aventurine. Effective for absorbing electromagnetic smog, this crystal defuses negative situations and turns them around. Place one at each corner of your desk or in the drawers, if you have a coworker who leaches your energy.
- Labradorite creates a harmonious working environment.
- Orange carnelian helps you to achieve maximum success and get things done as quickly as possible.
- Sodalite promotes good companionship and harmony between co-workers.
- Smoky quartz protects against others people stress and it alleviates communication difficulties. Keep one near your phone.

Crystal for energy healing within the body

The energy pathways are known as meridians, and the energy centers are known as chakras. The chakras are the areas of the highest density of energy and therefore are the easiest places to exchange energy with the outside world. Chakras go in and out of balance and alignment naturally, fluctuating with everyday highs and lows. The little stresses of life, minor illnesses, emotions, and even your thoughts, can change the equilibrium of your chakra system. When you are not feeling well for some time, your chakras go out of balance. Crystals are the best way to use for healing chakras.

Crystals for the base chakra

Location: Base of the spine
Color: Red
Crystal: Red jasper, red calcite, smoky quartz

Crystal for sacral chakra

Location: Just below the navel
Color: Orange
Crystal: Carnelian, orange calcite, copper

Crystal solar plexus chakra

> Location: Behind the soft cartilage at bottom of breastbone
> Color: yellow
> Crystal: Citrine, amber, tiger's eye, imperial topaz

Crystal for the heart chakra

> Location: Center of the chest
> Color: Green
> Crystal: Malachite, aventurine, jade, green moss agate

Crystal for throat chakra

> Location: Center of the throat
> Color: Blue
> Crystal: Blue lace, blue fluorite, aquamarine

Crystal for third eye

> Location: Above eyebrows
> Color: Indigo
> Crystal: Lapis lazuli, sodalite, moldavite

Crystal for crown chakra

> Location: Top of the head
> Color: Violet
> Crystal: amethyst, labradorite, selenite

Crystals work whenever they are around you. Crystals can aid in and promote so many aspects of your life. Once you start, you will find that you will add to your crystal collection regularly.

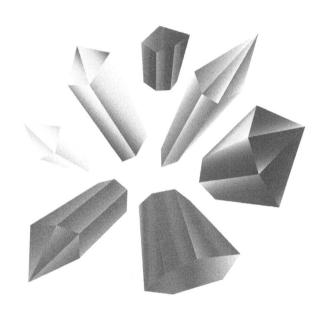

# Chapter 9

# Holistic Healing

*Our bodies are like rechargeable batteries using the earth and universe to recharge. The earth helps us to heal and gives us everything we need to survive and works with the universe to connect to a spiritual energy that keeps our bodies moving on a daily basis. Energetic healers believe that with the flow of energy, the body can heal itself naturally.*

We have a constant flow of energy from our feet to our minds. The physical body is purely a vehicle for the soul and the spirit. Treating one aspect in isolation from the others will lead to an incomplete cure, although on a physical level the patient may appear healed. When the body's energy flows freely and vitalized, the cells of the organs, tissues, blood, and bones are at an optimal level; and we are in perfect health.

Energy healing is a type of therapy that manipulates our physical energy circuits to help facilitate our body's healing mechanisms. This holistic approach is excellent for assisting in the healing process by unblocking our energy fields and helps to ward off future problems by identifying issues before they turn into pain within our physical body. Our bodies contain our histories—every chapter, line, and verse of every event and relationship in our lives. As our lives unfold, our biological health becomes a living breathing, biographical statement that conveys our strengths, weaknesses, hopes, and fears. When we carry emotional, mental, psychological, or spiritual energy, our bodies produce biological responses that are then stored in our cellular memory. In this way, our biographies are woven into our biological system gradually, slowly, every day. All physical health problems, emotional disturbances, and financial issues are related to energy blockage or imbalance. When people are experiencing major stressors in life, they can cause disruptions in the body and can lead to physical problems like insomnia and mood swings. More people are beginning to understand that they see positive changes by focusing on the healing of the body's energy.

The mind is a powerful thing and thoughts are directly connected to the energetic body and the physical body. One way to clear these energetic blockages is to let go of all past traumas and negative relationships. If you hold on to all of your negative experiences in life, then your body will respond in a negative way. So it is best to take each day as it comes, work through all of your emotions, and know you are a new you each day you wake up. By keeping your mind in balance, your body will follow.

Natural healing gives everyone the ability to improve themselves and lead a better life. When you are spiritually balanced, you are better able to stay positive and see life from a different point of view. This positive outlook takes away depression and allows the body to relax and maintain harmony before potential problems develop into energetic blockages.

In my studies, Lifeforce Energy Healing, by master healer and teacher Deborah King, I learned the path of how to heal yourself and to help others. There is the learning process involved in deepening your inner world, your consciousness. How do we strengthen our conscious minds and become more aware of the way our unconscious mind works? How do we transform old unhealthy ways of thinking and doing into more self-awareness? The pure self is pure consciousness. Here is deep inner security, no matter what is going on in your life. Here, right inside you, is the heart of your being. In the past, very few people made the journey to expanded consciousness into oneness. Now many of you are awakening. The global dilemmas that humanity is facing are at the root of a crisis of consciousness. The continued evolution of mankind on our planet, as well as our personal health and happiness, depends upon our ability to become more conscious. To learn about energy medicine, we have to know how energy works in the human body. The human energy field is organized into energy centers called chakras. Like the levels of your own energy field, these are centers of spinning energy that correspond to and affect different aspects in your life.

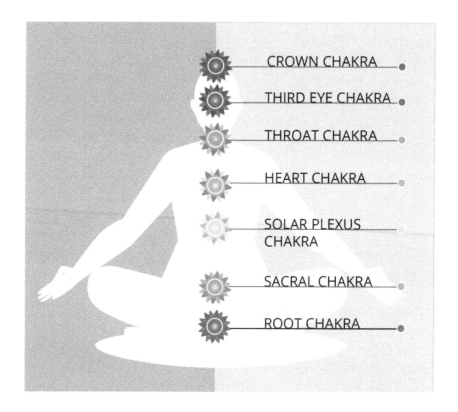

CROWN CHAKRA

THIRD EYE CHAKRA

THROAT CHAKRA

HEART CHAKRA

SOLAR PLEXUS CHAKRA

SACRAL CHAKRA

ROOT CHAKRA

## The Chakras

Chakra means "wheel of light" in Sanskrit, and each one looks a bit like a funnel or vortex that spins when it is operating optimally. As the chakras spin, there is a constant exchange of energy with the environment—going from them out into the world and the unified field coming in. The incoming energy nurtures and supports our individual energy field and physical bodies. These centers of spinning energy correspond to and heavily influence different aspects of your life. Like the levels of your field, the chakras are affected by your consciousness. If you get emotionally upset about something, these energy centers can become distorted or imbalanced. They can start spinning the wrong way. There are seven major chakras and more than twenty minor ones corresponding to the body. We focus on the seven main ones, which start at the base of the spine and run to the top of the head. The chakras are connected throughout you and to one another. When operating optimally, the current or path actually widens and allows more energy to flow through as you heighten consciousness and service to others. Our modern medical system also does not address the whole person, which often leaves us dissatisfied, even if unconsciously. It does not concentrate on the underlying causes of disease, and therefore it does not treat them, only the symptoms. This is one of the reasons why energy medicine is so valuable. It treats the body, including the psychological and spiritual dimensions as well. Let us see how chakras work.

The first root chakra

The root chakra is responsible for your sense of safety and security on the earthly journey. The root chakra is composed of whatever grounds you to stability in your life. This includes your basic needs such as food, water, shelter and safety, as well as your more emotional needs, such as letting go of fear. When these needs are met, you feel grounded and safe, and you tend to worry less.

Location: The base of the spine, the pelvic floor.

*Imbalances in the root chakra.* When there is an imbalance in the root chakra, you may experience anxiety disorders, fear, or nightmares. Physical imbalances may manifest as problems in the colon, with the bladder, with elimination or lower back, legs, or feet issues. In men, prostate problems may occur. Eating disorders may also be a sign of a root chakra imbalance.

*How to balance root chakra.* While meditation does connect you to a higher spiritual plane, it also serves to ground you. You may not always be able to trust that the world will give you what you need to survive. You are your own connection to your higher self and your trust in the power higher than yourself will give you what you need to feel safe.

For the best answer you have to ask questions for self-examination:

1. What belief pattern did you inherit from your family?
2. Which of those belief patterns that still have authority in your thinking can you acknowledge are no longer valid?
3. Do you have a personal code of honor? What is it?
4. Have you ever compromised your sense of honor? If so, have you taken steps to heal it?
5. Do you have any unfinished business with our family members? If so, list the reason that prevents you from healing your family relationships.
6. List all the blessings that you feel came from your family.
7. If you are now raising a family of your own, list the qualities that you would like your children to learn from you.
8. What traditions and rituals do you continue for yourself and your family?
9. Describe the characteristics within yourself that you would like to strengthen and develop.

Root chakra balance is so important to connect with Mother Nature, to walk barefoot on the grass, to hug a tree, and answer all questions above.

Second chakra: the power of relationships

The second chakra is the partnership chakra. Its energy begins to pulsate and become distinct around the age of seven. At that age, children start interacting with other children and adults, more independently of their parents and outside the home environment. Through these initial interactions they begin to individuate, form relationships, and explore their power of choice.

Location: Lower abdomen to navel area.

Energy connection to physical: sexual organs, large intestine, lower vertebrae, pelvis, hip area, appendix, and bladder. Energy connection to the emotional/mental body: This chakra resonates to our need for relationships with other people and our need to control to some extent the dynamics of our physical environment.

*Key issues.* When the second chakra is imbalanced, it can create urinary or bladder issues, chronic low back pain, inflammatory bowel disease, colitis, and Crohn's disease. Addiction is a very common problem for people with sacral chakra distortions. Since the second chakra is where your pleasure sensors lie, it is easy to get trapped in an unbalanced sacral chakra and become addicted to whatever gives you relief from your problems, worries, or emotions. This can include drugs, alcohol, and food addictions, but also behaviors like gambling, excessive shopping, or surfing the Internet and sexual escapes like pornography. Nearly everyone on the planet has second chakra issues, so you are not alone. Energy healing will help you uncover the underlying emotional causes of an unbalanced second chakra.

*Healing your second chakra.* Touch is vitally important for healing the second chakra. Without touch, we are "out of touch" with ourselves and with others. A hug, a massage, holding your pet—any type of gentle touch brings harmony. The second chakra is happy in water, so swimming or bathing can boost the health of your sacral chakra. To help balance and charge this chakra and express your creativity, surround yourself with beauty, particularly sweet-smelling flowers, and use the essential oils of musk or sandalwood.

The third chakra: personal power

Third chakra energy, the energy of the personal power chakra, becomes the dominant vibration in our development during puberty. It assists us further in the process of individuation, of forming a "self" ego and personality separate from our inherited identity. This energy center also contains most issues related to the development of personal power and self-esteem. The third chakra completes the physical trilogy of the human energy system.

Location: the solar plexus

Energy connection to the emotional/mental body: stomach, pancreas, adrenals, upper intestines, gallbladder, liver, and the middle spine, located behind the solar plexus.

What can happen when the third chakra is not operating correctly?

- Problems with the pancreas (including diabetes and hypoglycemia)
- Digestive problems, including ulcer
- Liver problems, including cirrhosis, hepatitis, and liver cancer
- Hiatal hernia
- Gallstones
- Varicose veins
- Problems with the spleen

Third chakra balance shows itself as one who is responsible, with good self-discipline, someone who is confident and energetic, has some playful moments, and is able to take risks. Take a moment at the end of every day and note whether or not you meditated, journaled, exercised, or had other personal care. By taking the time to reflect, you are building your willpower. Remember, don't criticize yourself if you missed an item. Simply resolve to make time the next day. This is the best way to build an effective will.

The fourth chakra: emotional power

The fourth chakra is the central powerhouse of the human energy system. The middle chakra, it mediates between the body and spirit and determines their health and strength. Fourth chakra energy is emotional in nature and helps propel our emotional development. This chakra embodies the spiritual lesson that teaches us how to act out of love and compassion and recognize that the most powerful energy we have is love.

Location: center of the chest

Energy connection to the physical body: heart and circulatory system, ribs, breast, thymus gland, lungs, shoulders, arms, hands, and diaphragm. Energy connection to the emotional/mental body: This chakra resonates to our emotional perceptions, which determine the quality of our lives far more than our mental perceptions. As children, we react to our circumstance with a range of emotions: love, compassion, hope, despair, hate, envy, and fear. As adults, we are challenged to generate within ourselves an emotional climate and steadiness from which to act consciously and with compassion.

This chakra is all about balance, within ourselves and with our relationships and our environment. Self-love is an important component in being able to reach this state of balance. We can't truly love someone if we don't love ourselves first. This requires an understanding and acceptance of our dualities. The fourth chakra rules over the heart, lungs, pericardium, thymus, upper back, ribs, arms, and hands. Conditions of a distorted heart chakra can include problems with the heart and circulatory system. It also could manifest itself as a disorder of the lungs, including lung cancer, pneumonia, bronchitis, emphysema, breast cancer, and breast disorders such as mastitis or cysts, immune system deficiencies, asthma, or shortness of breath or allergies.

*How to heal your heart chakra.* Loving and being loved is your birthright. An open and compassionate heart is the result of a balanced heart chakra. Get a pet to love! Pets love us unconditionally, making it safe for us to learn to love again. Search out the roots of your consciousness that may be telling you there is no hope of your experiencing real love. Meditate and journal, journal and meditate. Make the intention to be open to loving yourself and others more. Work to soften any walls you have erected around your heart. Listen to your body, mind, and heart to find out what works best for you. By doing what you love, you will be rewarded with love in return.

The fifth chakra

The fifth chakra embodies the challenges of surrendering our own willpower and spirits to the will of a higher power. From a spiritual perspective, our highest goal is the full release of our personal will into the "hands of the divine."

Location: the throat

Energy connection to the physical body: throat, thyroid, trachea, esophagus, parathyroid, hypothalamus, neck vertebrae, mouth, jaw, and teeth. Energy connection to the emotional/mental body: the fifth chakra resonates to the numerous emotional and mental struggles involved in learning the nature of the power of choice. All illness has a connection to the fifth chakra because choice is involved in every detail of our lives and therefore in every illness.

When this area is out of balance, the follow conditions can arise:

- Any disorder of the voice, mouth, teeth, or gums
- Tight neck and other neck problems
- Swollen glands in the throat, sore throat, throat cancer
- Chronic sinus problems
- Joint disorder in the jaw
- Thyroiditis, thyroid cancer

To evaluate the health of your throat chakra, you want to ask yourself, am I honest with myself and take responsibility for my own personal needs?

*How to balance your fifth chakra.* Begin writing all of your thoughts, feelings, and insight about yourself in a personal journal. Use it daily or hourly, if you need to. Clear the energy in this chakra through speech or the emission of sound. You may need to take it up a notch and yell or scream. Just remember to do it safely, in a mindful way that does not hurt yourself or others, remembering that healing is rarely about confrontation. Take singing lessons or participate in group singing. Sing as much as you can. Chanting works as well. Let yourself go into a state of creativity using dance, voice, writing, drawing, and/or painting. Open yourself to receive guidance, solutions, and success.

The sixth chakra: the power of mind

The sixth chakra involves our mental and reasoning abilities and our psychological skill at evaluating our beliefs and attitudes. The mind chakra resonates to the energies of our psyches, our conscious and unconscious psychological forces. Within eastern spiritual literature, the sixth chakra is the "third eye," the spiritual center in which the interaction of mind and psyche can lead to intuitive sight and wisdom. This is the chakra of wisdom. The sixth chakra is concerned with opening the mind, developing an impersonal mind and learning to act on internal direction.

Location: center of forehead

Energy connection to the physical body: The brain and neurological system, pituitary and pineal glands, as well as the eyes, ears, and nose. Energy connection to the emotional/mental body: the sixth chakra links us to our mental body, our intelligence, and psychological characteristics. Our psychological characteristics are a combination of what we know and what we believe to be true, a combination of the facts, fears, personal experiences, and memories that are active within our mental energy body.

*Third-eye chakra: key issues.* The third eye chakra governs what we see, what we imagine, and what we psychically and intuitively perceive. It's also associated with memory and dreams; so when the sixth chakra is unbalanced, we can have nightmares, hallucinations, or memory concentration difficulties. This energy center rules the eyes, nose, brain, neurological system and pineal gland. So when it is imbalanced or blocked, we can suffer from eye problems, sinus, headaches, stroke, and neurological disturbances. People are often empathic and absorb a lot of energy from others. Turn off electronics, unplug the phone, light candles, and just be. Solitude is a way to replenish yourself. Visually pleasing environments also help to heal this chakra. Use light colors. Try the scents of sandalwood, star anise, gardenia, lavender, and rosemary. Try crystal therapy using a purple amethyst.

The seventh chakra: our spiritual connector

The seventh chakra is our connection to our spiritual nature and our capacity to allow our spirituality to become an integral part of our physical lives and guide us. While our energy system as a whole is animated by our spirit, the seventh chakra is directly aligned to seek an intimate relation with the divine. It is the chakra of prayer. It's also the warehouse for the energy we amass through kind thoughts and actions, and through acts of faith and prayer.

Location: top of the head

Energy connection to the physical body: the seventh chakra is the entry point for the human life force, which pours endlessly into the human energy system, from the greater universe, from the divine. The energy of the seventh chakra influences that of the major body systems: the central nervous system, the muscular system, and the skin.

Energy connection to the emotional/mental body: the seventh chakra contains the energy that generates devotion, inspirational and prophetic thoughts, transcendent ideas, and mystical connections.

*Key issues.* Your seventh chakra creates your belief system, your perception, and the world through thought. If your belief system was created in the wake of a trauma, you may operate from a place of fear or mistrust, which colors everything you experience and can affect your quality of life. Physically, the seventh chakra connects to your brain, pineal and pituitary glands, and central nervous system. Imbalances in the seventh chakra can cause headaches, strokes, brain tumors, epilepsy, Parkinson's, and Alzheimer's diseases.

Seventh chakra archetypes: egotist and sage

The egotist is proud, self-important, narcissistic, and believes only they are responsible for their accomplishments. The functional archetype, the sage, knows that they are ones with the spirit and embodies love and awareness. The chakra system is a powerful diagnostic tool. Chakra imbalances manifest themselves as a physical feeling of tension or pain in the area where the chakra lies. It is a useful tipoff to what is going on in your energy field. Once you know which chakra can use healing, you become empowered to work on the energetic level to heal mind, body, and spirit. When I took the course of chakra wisdom by Deborah King, I learned some tools on how to balance the chakras.

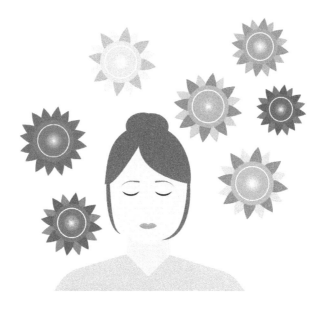

Meditation for balancing chakras

Meditation is one of the most effective ways to balancing the chakras. Begin by sitting with your eyes closed in the traditional lotus position. It is okay to meditate while sitting in a chair too, as long as you keep your back straight. Focus on grounding yourself to the earth via your root chakra. Feel the natural energy of the earth radiating though your body. Once your intuition tells you that you are sufficiently grounded, you can begin opening each chakra. Starting from the root and working your way up, visualize each chakra as a flower of the appropriate color—a red flower for the root chakra and an orange flower for the sacral chakra, etc. (You can find all the correct colors on page 133). Visualize the flower blooming. This practice will open your chakras and help you to work through blockages and imbalances. Try to spend about four to six minutes or more visualizing each chakra. Continue your chakra balancing meditation throughout your week, or as needed. Just remember to always listen to them. The most important outcome of your meditating for 20 minutes twice a day is that you are helping every sentient being on the planet. When you hear something bad on the news, see devastating images on your TV or computer screen, or you worry about whatever is bothering you—go meditate. It is important to remember that when meditating, you should only focus on one thing at a time. Usually, the mind tries to hold several different thoughts and ideas at once. When you sit down to meditate for the first time, you realize how cluttered the mind is. However, the mind can be tamed and forced to concentrate on a single thought.

Another way to learn concentration is through the use of a mantra. A *mantra* is the repetition of a sacred word. For example, you might repeat the mantra *aum* a certain number of times. Repeating a mantra forces the mind to focus on single thought. After you have practiced concentration and learned to focus on one thing at a time, you can proceed to the next stage with no thoughts at all. Achieving a silent mind is difficult, but when you attain it, the experience is really unique and powerful.

Through meditation, you attain the power to control your thoughts and on occasion stop them completely. It takes time and practice. Meditation is a simple and spontaneous action. Our mind is used to complication, and it takes time to forget bad habits. There are so many amazing benefits of meditation, like providing the nervous system a rest five times deeper than sleep. It's possible to let go of the stress we have all accumulated throughout life.

Guidelines for meditation

1. Sit comfortably with your back straight. You want to be relaxed, but not falling asleep. Don't lie down or slump on a couch. You'll need something to support your back so that your posture remains erect but without your body having to strain.
2. Close your eyes. Always meditate with your eyes closed.
3. Intend to meditate for approximately twenty minutes. Don't use an alarm or any other device that will jolt you awake quickly. It takes about a couple weeks, sometimes more, but pretty soon you'll have a sense of time. If at first you need some help, just place a clock nearby and peek at it from time to time.
4. When the twenty minutes are up, keep your eyes closed for two to five minutes before opening your eyes and going back to your day. Otherwise, the abrupt shift from one state of consciousness—the meditative state to the working state may give you a headache.
5. Meditate for twenty minutes twice a day—once in the morning and once in the late afternoon or early evening.

Stress, energy, and healthy living

Since my life was affected by World War II, I grew up with less food leading to high levels of stress. I became very ill. I was paralyzed at the age of five on the left side of my body. At the age of ten, I developed tuberculosis. At the age of twelve, I was diagnosed with an infection of the gallbladder and was prescribed many medications. The medications had many side effects and led to low energy levels. I sensed that there was a healthier way of living. I worked very hard to educate myself. I wanted to understand what were the wholesome foods leading to nutritional balance and a healthy lifestyle. I also continued my formal studies culminating in graduating with a doctorate in agricultural science. I then continued my studies in alternative medicine, but still felt that I needed more knowledge so I continued my coursework learning more about the healing powers of energy. I came to the conclusion that everything is energy; and I leveraged my knowledge and beliefs to find strength, energy, and balance in my life.

## My Master Class with Deborah King

As a child, my life was affected by World War II, when my family lived under Soviet Union control and under the German Nazi regime. Growing up in unsanitary conditions, along with the stress of not having enough food for long periods of time, caused me to become very physically and emotionally ill. Although there were not many educated people at the time in my country, I had a vision that getting an education would bring happiness to my life. I worked extremely hard, and I eventually earned a PhD in agriculture science. I became a successful business woman in Lithuania, but I continued to feel that my life was not in harmony. I knew how to handle stressful situations, but I was still unhappy most of the time. My work as a scientist at the Institute in Lithuania taught me to understand the great importance of organic food in a human's life. The quality of the production of plants is directly dependent on our actions. My focus during my earlier life was science-based, and I knew little about the great effect of spirituality in my life. The master class with Deborah King unlocked my powerful healing nature. It allowed me to remove energy blockages and to adjust the energy flow of the endocrine system, bringing the body into balance and harmony. I learned to push away pain, anxiety, and negative emotions. Thanks to Deborah King's master class, the clouds and stormy days are over. "Healing is the end of conflict with yourself," says Stephanie Gailing.

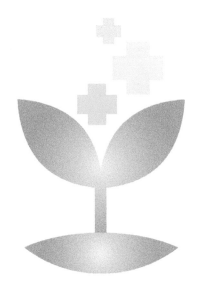

# Chapter 10

# Creating a Lifestyle Plan

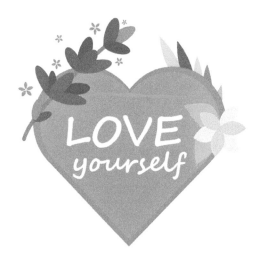

### Self-Love

Nobody is perfect. We all make mistakes. We all struggle to like ourselves. Self-love will take you where you want to go in life and will help you work toward your goals. Self-love is the answer to becoming successful. I found that there is only one thing that heals every problem, and that is to know how to love yourself. I used to think that loving yourself is selfish, but it is not! Caring about ourselves will make it easier to love others and will help us to take care of the environment around us. We can really help the planet when we come from a space of great love and joy on an individual basis. We are in charge of our lives. If you are not willing to love yourself today, then you are not going to love yourself tomorrow because whatever excuse you had today, you will still have it tomorrow and the same excuse ten years later. When you practice self-love, you are continually naming and claiming all of who you are, even the scariest parts. It is about developing your capacity to be aware, authentic, and intentional in every aspect of your life. In doing so, you build greater self-compassion and enhance your ability to offer compassion to others. While self-love is a lifelong practice, Liz DiAlto of the Institute of Integrative Nutrition (IIN) suggests that we can build a healthy foundation by practicing five principles:

1. Acceptance
2. Respect
3. Awareness
4. Knowledge
5. Trust

Acceptance

Acceptance takes work. Be gentle with yourself. Accept things that happened without worry and judgment. Forgive and leave behind all toxic activities that will not serve you anymore. Change your self-talk. Replace the phrase "I am not good enough" with more positive messages such as the following:

- *My life is a gift.*
- *I am good enough.*
- *I love myself deeply and fully.*
- *I am worthy of love.*
- *I am talented.*

Surround yourself with positive people who will help you bring the best out in you. Release negative thoughts and embrace positivity and optimism. Write down positive statements about yourself. Affirmations can help us handle our negative feelings about ourselves.

They help increase self-reliance and help you take action with life and build self-confidence. They even increase your self-esteem. When you repeat an affirmation over and over again, it begins to seep into your brain that the affirmation is true. This helps you re-affirm your internal positive thinking and gradually chases away your negativity.

Respect

One of the best ways to respect yourself is to never settle for less than you deserve. You deserve the best in life. You have but one life to live. Don't settle for less than the best. To achieve this, you must forgive yourself for past mistakes. Letting go of the past can be difficult, but in order to respect who you are now, you must let go of who you were then. You can never look back. You must move forward with positivity. Work on building your confidence. Do things you are good at. Accept compliments, and make note of when others are proud of you. Honesty is the ultimate respect. Even when it is hard, the truth is always the way to go. Surround yourself with positive people. This means that you are keeping company with those that respect you while avoiding those that make you feel bad about yourself.

Awareness

Before you can make changes in yourself you have to examine your strengths and faults. Becoming self-aware is the process of understanding yourself. Emotional awareness means being able to recognize emotions that you experience; understand the feelings associated with the emotion and what you think and do as a result of those emotions. Athletes get intensive training in how to overcome negative emotions. When you are aware of your strengths and weaknesses, you will become more confident in what you do. Awareness of self can be developed. Spend some time recognizing areas you need to develop and intentionally make an effort to strengthen your weaknesses.

Write down your strengths, and ask others that you trust to give you advice. Value your beliefs and principles of your life. Knowing your values is an essential part of building awareness of yourself. Being supportive of others is probably the most endearing quality you can integrate into your personality.

Knowledge

Knowledge is a familiarity, awareness, or understanding of someone or something. It can be facts, information, or skills that are acquired through direct experience. Firsthand experience is a powerful and practical type of knowledge. You can also acquire knowledge by study, reading books, or attending classes. Knowledge is the most powerful force in the universe. The good news is that you are surrounded by knowledge from the Internet, books, libraries, and universities. The bad news is that you have to be hungry for that knowledge. Thomas Friedman called it curiosity quotient (CQ).

Recognize that who you are in any moment can change. Give yourself permission to be someone different today than you were yesterday. Clarify your core values. Get to know yourself better by considering what your top values are. For example: expressing yourself creatively, connecting with your community, being healthy and having financial stability.

Trust

Self-trust means that you can take care of your needs and safety. It means you trust yourself to survive situations and practice kindness, not perfection. When you fail to fulfill your own promises due to lack of willpower, you find it difficult to trust yourself. You may have conflicting goals or lack of determination to follow your goals. How do you learn to trust yourself? Start by avoiding people who undermine your self-trust. Think about the people around you. Do they have the same goals and ethics as you do? Do you really want them in your life? Keep promises to yourself. Developing self-trust also includes becoming your own best friend. Making a commitment and keeping it builds trust in yourself. For instance, you could make a commitment to walk every day or to stop eating junk food every day. Learn to walk your talk and fulfill your promises to trust yourself and become a trustworthy person. Believe that you are safe to express yourself in a bolder way than the way you did in the past even if others do not fully approve. Listen to your physical body. Trust that your body is always sending important signals. "It is safe for me to be me. It is safe for me to be here."

## Relationships

Relationships fill our world. They are inescapable. Whether we are in relationships with a spouse, children, extended family members, coworkers, bosses, friends, neighbors, or even strangers, we are challenged to learn how to get along. Strong, positive relationships don't just happen. They require time, attention, understanding and a willingness to see that the needs of the other person are as important as our own needs. Our relationships, from close family, to coworkers, bosses, employees, and others, whom we regularly interact with, mark our path and is an important part of our lives.

My family had a difficult time surviving after World War II. As a child, I did not get as much love as I needed. My father was killed in the war, and my mother had to work to provide food for the family. After my mother remarried, I had three brothers to help to take care of. I was abused by my stepfather. After thirty-eight years of married life, I had a loving time with my husband. He used to repeat, "No one in the world loves you like I do." I did not believe him. I thought everyone that is married would love their spouse.

I had so many questions from people. What secret did I use to keep the family so strong? The answer is respect for one another. Respect is the foundation for creating honesty, trust, friendship, and love for your partner. To put it simply, respect your partner the way you want them to respect you. If you don't have respect for your partner and your mental and physical well-being, how do you expect to thrive as a couple? You must accept and not judge each other. Everyone has a past and has made mistakes or has a different opinion. You must support and encourage each other without judgment.

A loving relationship is about lifting each other up and not tearing them down. Strong communication is important. When I could not go on vacation at the same time as my husband, I used to go to the health spa for two weeks by myself. My husband always sent me a post card every day. Yes, every day! I usually make a phone call to ask him about his day. No relationship can survive without open and honest communication. When communication begins to break down, it often signals the relationship is breaking down as well. You need to have faith in each other.

One of the vital aspects of a successful relationship is to have faith in each other. This will keep the relationship secure, stable, and will last a lifetime. Trust your partner. It is also important to remember if you truly trust each other, when your partner wants to go out with his friends, there will be no issue. Partners who lack trust usually are projecting their own insecurities.

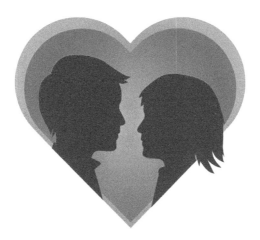

Relationships with children

Good family relationships help your children feel secure and loved. They help you feel good too! Creating a family that runs smoothly is a work in progress. This is taking numerous small steps to form long-term results. Our family expends more love with the birth of each child. We worked hard to protect our children from outside negativities and kept our children close to us. We had our own model on how to raise the children. Building a life together takes a lot more than love. Internalize these points and invest in your relationship to have a happily ever after. In my family, we have these family rules:

1. Treat each other with respect.
2. Help each other at all times.
3. Work together to solve problems.
4. Play together.
5. Do not bully one another.

Teamwork and family relationships

When your family is working as a team, everyone feels supported and is able to contribute. It is easier to work as a team when everyone knows where they stand. We shared the housework. I did the meal planning and cooking. My son did the vacuuming, and my husband took out the garbage and did the food shopping.

My daughter cleaned the kitchen. Everyone had to make their own bed in the morning. We had a garden outside of the city, and we all enjoyed planting and taking care of the plants. We enjoyed eating fresh vegetables, berries, and fruit. My children learned to take care of themselves and to eat healthy food. My youngest son became a vegetarian. My sons learned how to do handy work around the house. We learned that good communication was more effective when it became spontaneous rather than formulaic. A speech that is read rarely has more impact than a speech that is delivered spontaneously. We used positive communication in the family and avoided speaking words of anger or frustration as much as possible.

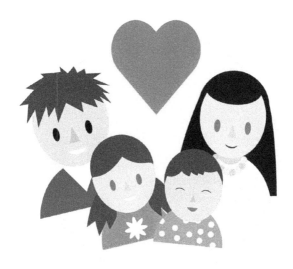

How to improve relationships

1. Your relationships reflect the relationship you have with yourself. Take responsibility for your own happiness. Treat yourself with care, acceptance, and gentle compassion.
2. Everyone wants to know that you care about them. Show them that you care.
3. Positive thoughts and deeds inspire others' respect and cause them to value the relationship.
4. When the relationship is tested, practice forgiveness and learn to forgive.
5. Keep stress in check. How many times have you felt stressed when you have a disagreement with your spouse, kids, boss, friends, or coworkers and then said or did something you later regretted. If you can quickly relieve stress and return to a calm state, you'll not only avoid such regrets; but in many cases, you will also help to calm the other person as well.
6. Avoid negative body language. If you disagree with or dislike what is being said, you might use negative body language to rebuff the other person's message, such as crossing your arms, avoiding eye contact, or tapping your feet. You

don't have to agree with everything, but to communicate effectively, it is important to avoid sending negative signals.

7. You need to learn to understand people. If you desire to improve your understanding of people so that you can build positive relationships, then keep in mind the following truths about people and actions you can take to bridge the gap often caused by them.

8. You will enjoy life more if you like people. Think about the people that you have known for a moment. When have you known someone with the positive characteristics who live life and have a lot of fun? If you like people, then no matter where you go, you will meet a friend.

More about relationships

The most important thing in a relationship is connection. Connection is the feeling of being on the same team, of understanding each other, that inexplicable warm feeling of being in love. When you feel connected and united in your relationship, as if by magic, everything including your communication will begin to flow much more easily and effortlessly. Do not look for happiness from others. This is an unreliable source of happiness. Others do not fill our emotional needs, "If you do not love yourself entirely and actively ensure your own needs are met, you will find it difficult to do the same for others." We have to learn to fix our own problems. We only control ourselves—we do not control other people. We have to focus on taking responsibility. Love and responsibility for yourself will open the door to your future.

Reach your goals

Personal goals can provide long-term direction and short-term motivation. Goals help us put focus on what we want to be and where we want to go with our lives. They can be a way of utilizing knowledge and managing time and resources so that you can focus on making the most of your life's potential. Goals give you a direction to move forward and inspire you to keep moving. Each goal gives you clarity. Your goals taken together give you a way to assess your progress in life.

Remember your goals must be your own. The goals you pick should be ones you care about. They should be important to you. Make your goals specific, about what you want to accomplish. When you think about your future, do not be afraid to dream big. When you hit an obstacle, it won't stop you because your eyes are set on the bigger prize.

Write your story

Write down in a one or two-page article the story of your desired future. Write down what you will be doing, where you will be living, how you will enjoy your success. Your future may be forgotten before you had a chance to work on it. Make your goal specific because this has a greater chance of success. Visualize how to achieve your goals. Learn how to achieve your goals with the power of creative dreaming. That's it! Now you know how to visualize. Vitalize your goal for at least five minutes. Do this at least once a day. For speedy results, visualize as often as you would like. Just do what feels right for you.

Another visualization technique is to create a photograph or picture of yourself as if your goals were already achieved. If one of your goals is to own a new car, take your camera down to your local auto dealer. Have a picture taken of you sitting behind the wheel of your dream car. If your dream is to visit Italy, then find a poster of Rome or Venice, cut out a picture of yourself and paste it onto the picture of your dream city. Create a picture or visual representation of every goal you have. It can be a financial goal, career, or learning a new skill. Visualizing involves creating images, whether it be in your mind or physically creating them. This shows you your goals and dreams that you have in life. Visualization helps you find, manifest, and focus on your goals and aspirations. Once you have the images and visions in your mind, you can start to feel emotions you have for your goals as well. This can help to motivate you and help you to continue trying to achieve these goals. The most important part of the visualization is your emotions and feelings. You must absolutely induce feelings into your vision. Feelings give life to your inner vision and start the growth of your goals into material form. The more detailed is your vision, the easier it will be for you to awaken the feelings.

## Learn to Be Positive

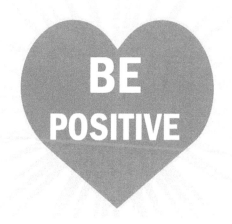

So many people do not believe that they can achieve their goals. Why? Because they think that life is tough and things are difficult. These are all limiting beliefs that will destroy your plan. If you have such a negative thought and negative beliefs about your abilities, you won't be able to achieve your goals. You are shooting yourself in the foot! If you have a negative belief about something, your reality will represent that belief, and you will continue to believe it because you think it is true. You must find ways to reorient all your thoughts to be positive—by reading books, seeking professional help, talking to friends, taking walks, and going to the gym. Surround yourself with positive and enthusiastic people. Whenever you get stuck in a negative spiral, you should have people to talk to, who can put everything in perspective rather than feed your negative thinking. Make a list of the things you are grateful for at the moment. Your list may include things like your health, pets, relationships, or even a new yoga class. Add anything you consider to be relevant. Read motivational and positive material. Remind yourself that nobody is perfect and allow yourself to make mistakes. The best and only thing you can do is to learn from your errors and move forward.

# Find Clarity

Look deep inside yourself. That is where the answers are. Deepak Chopra recommends "to examine your reality in here, which is where clarity can be found." There are many actions you can take and make mental adjustments. You can make moves that will help you shift from uncertainty to certainty.

1. Take responsibility for your own level of clarity.
2. Clarity is not something that arrives from outside of you. Clarity is not a matter of luck. Clarity is what you create for yourself.
3. Clarity is a decision, when you commit yourself to one specific direction.
4. Clarity is the natural result.
5. If you want more clarity, then it is time to treat the generation of clarity as a serious undertaking that is 100 percent your responsibility.
6. It is not going to happen unless you make it happen.

Clarity-boosting patterns

Focused people are those who can tell you their purpose and direction. You need to feed your mind with inspiration and motivational material like quality books and audio programs. You need to eat healthy unrefined foods, especially fruits and vegetables, fresh juices and smoothies. This will help keep your mind sharp and alert. Avoid stimulants because they can cause mood swings in your thoughts and emotions.

The lessons on clarity from your past show you that your level of clarity is not the same at all times. Take a moment to review those times when you identify some factors that can increase your clarity.

## Explore and Experiment

Sometimes it is tough to set a clear goal because you do not know what you are getting into. As a gardener, I experimented with growing flowers and vegetables. As a health coach, I realized that food is not the only way for the healthy body. We need good relationships. Love, body, mind, and spirit must work together. For this reason, you have to get moving first before clarity can be achieved.

To define your strengths, ask yourself some questions:

1. What do I enjoy doing the most? What is the biggest success that I ever had?
2. How would I describe my ideal job? What was my favorite job, and what did I like about it?
3. If I could have any job at all, anywhere, what would it be?
4. If I won a million dollars in the lottery and had to pick a job to work at indefinitely, what would I choose to do with my time?
5. What activities energize me?

Then make a list of goals and put them in order of importance to you right now. If this goal is truly important, you should center your life around it.

## Take Control

In reality, you are completely in charge of your product, quality control, training, development, and finances. You give yourself opportunities in the final analysis. No one but you can make the critical decisions for your future and your fortune. Be in control of your life. Be the master of yourself and sit in the driver's seat. You must have a plan and take action.

## Emotional Growth and Development

Setting goals help you organize your time. If you want to get to your dream and get to these goals that help you grow, you need to have some skills.

- Communication skills
  This will help you communicate your thoughts.

- Problem solving skills
  This will help you make decisions and solve problems.

- Self-confidence
  If you don't believe in yourself, your skills and abilities, then you can't expect anyone else to believe in you.

- Public speaking
  Public speaking is a very crucial skill to have. It requires a lot of self-confidence, practice, and analyzing of your audience.

- Sales and marketing
  The knowledge of the principles and methods of promoting, presenting, and selling products. Knowledge of at least the basics in marketing strategy, as well as a range of sales techniques, may come in handy.

- Computer and electronic skills.
  As we move to rely more on technology to help us conduct our daily tasks, we need to understand circuit boards, processors, electronic equipment, and computers.

## Spirituality

"Religion is belief in someone else's experience. Spirituality is having your own experience," according to Deepak Chopra. To be spiritual means to rise above the temptations of the body and the senses to realize the final Truth. To be religious means to observe rituals and rites. All religions have specific rituals and rites. This is not against religions. They all have their own purpose.

Spirituality is a broad concept with room for many perspectives. In general, it includes a sense of connection to something bigger than yourself, which can result in positive emotions, such as peace, contentment, gratitude, and acceptance. Spiritual well-being is cultivating a positive state of mind that incorporates a connection to something larger than yourself.

There are no rules to spirituality. It encourages you to listen to your intuition and do what is right for yourself and others around you. It truly sets you free to be the best you can and to be a good person with no promise of punishment or reward. The reward is your own inner happiness. Spirituality is based on love, not fear. You focus all of your energy into only the good and to act only based on love. This is a key point for me as any choice made out of fear will not be good for your soul. Spirituality sees the truth and focuses on the quality of the divine message about punishment or the threat of hell. Spirituality only speaks about karma. It is the law of attraction: you get what you give. Simple spirituality reminds us that we are not separate.

There are no borders, no racial differences, and no cultural divides. Like your sense of purpose, your personal definition of spiritual may change throughout your life, adapting to your own experiences and relationships. Spirituality means to return to that natural state of self where we are just beings without a shade of artificiality in us. When we start thinking and stay aware of our natural state, we start becoming spiritual.

Many spiritual traditions have a long history of using contemplative practices to increase compassion and empathy, as well as to quiet the mind. Having a strong spiritual outlook may help you find the meaning of life's difficult circumstances. Spiritual people make healthier choices and live longer.

# Intuition

Intuition is a connection to the Creator of the universe or your soul, all waiting patiently for your instruction and more than happy to guide you. So why don't humans just have gold rolling out over every home, happy relationships, and eternal good health? We have forgotten how to communicate such things to the universe. Intuition is a "knowing" that is not explained by facts or thoughts but through a deep inner feeling. It is "I feel it in my gut." Or it is "something doesn't feel quite right." Intuition is only about the present. There is no worrying about past or future.

"Intuition does not tell you what you want to hear, it tell you what you need to hear," said Sonia Chaquette-Tully, spiritual teacher and consultant. Our intuition offers the opportunity to bring awareness to the seemingly small choices that shape our life experiences. You already access your intuition on a daily basis. You tap into guidance from your higher self and spirit guides all the time. At the subconscious level, you already have intimate, familiar guidance managing routine things in the collective consciousness. Most people unfortunately only turn to their intuition when faced with uncertainty around a major life decision. Your body is not conditioned to take on such a challenge. When you train for a marathon, you begin with running only short distances. Similarly, the best place to start applying your intuition is with life's smaller choices, where your emotional investment is not so high.

Joel Pearson, from the University of New South Wales, Australia, has studied intuition and has concluded that there is evidence that intuition exists. His study showed that information was subconsciously perceived in the brain and helped with decisions. Pearson and colleagues found that people were able to make faster and more accurate decisions when they unconsciously were shown emotional images by a technique called continuous flash suppression. Those given these emotional images were able to process and utilize information from the images to improve their decisions. The HeartMath Institute in Australia has an extensive collection of materials on intuition. They recommend using the EM wave or Inner Balance technology to help enhance spiritual and self-growth techniques. The feel this intuition energy carries messages and information into a field environment that is shared by and connects everyone. In other words, we are all connected and are part of the field, an intelligent field of universal consciousness.

Intuition is a brilliant thing. The sharper it is, the better off you will be. Here are some pieces advice of how to tune in and sharpen your intuition:

1. Listen to the sound. Your intuition can speak to you. You start to take notice. Just try it.
2. Trust your gut feeling. Research suggests that emotions and intuition have a physical presence. This is the "sick feeling" about having to make a tough decision or knowing that a decision was a bad one.
3. Feel. You will feel it in your belly, and you will have goose bumps on your skin, and maybe even a shiver down your spine. Your heart will race, and you will quicken your breath.
4. Let bad feelings go. Negative emotions will cloud intuition, which is why when you are angry or depressed, you are more likely to make bad decisions.
5. Avoid negative people. Keep people who enrich and empower you. Walk away from those who drain you.
6. Try exercises to develop your intuition.

## Forgiveness

"Forgiveness is the only way to heal," says Don Miguel Ruiz, author of *The Four Agreements*. Forgiveness means different things to different people. The act that hurts you might always be with you, but forgiveness can lessen its grip on you and help free you from the control of the person who harmed you. We might forgive too quickly to avoid pain or to manipulate the situation. Forgiveness can release the pain and frees us from focusing on the other person. We have to be careful not to simply cover our wounds and delay the healing process. Forgiveness helps you achieve even your most practical and immediate goals. Perhaps you want a better job or to earn more money. You may want to have better relationships or live in a nicer place. Forgiveness helps you achieve all of these. Every aspect of your life will change for the better as you learn to forgive. Learning to forgive will improve all your relationships because your attitude will improve.

If you want to move up to the next level of financial abundance and success, forgiveness will help you achieve it. Forgiveness helps you heal not only your emotional scars but your physical ones too! The Mayo Clinic looked at the health implications of letting go of grudges and resentments. They found that forgiveness led to healthier relationships, less anxiety, less stress and hostility, and greater spiritual and physiological well-being. It also improved the immune system, heart health, and self-esteem. As you forgive and let go, your life will no longer be defined by your pain. You will have a greater compassion and understanding toward others.

How to forgive

Forgiveness requires will to forgive. Sometimes you cannot because the pain went too deep or the person was too abusive. If you decide you are willing to forgive, find a good place and time to be alone with your thoughts. Accept how you felt about it and how it made you react. You need to acknowledge the reality of what occurred and how you were affected. Acknowledge what you learned about yourself and how you grew from that event. Now think about how the other person acted because of his limited beliefs. Decide what you want to tell the other person about forgiveness. If you decide not to express forgiveness directly, do it on your own. Say the words "I forgive you" out loud and explain how you feel.

Express yourself

If the relationship is important to you, it may be very useful for you to tell the other person how their actions affected you. If that person is no longer in your life, if you want to cut off the relationship, you may want to write it in a letter and then tear up the letter or burn it and move on. It will help put your feelings into perspective and become part of the letting-go process. Give yourself permission to do it right. When you find yourself focusing on a past offense, you can say these words, "Thank you universe for this reminder of how important forgiveness is." Best ways to let go of a painful past:

1.   Make the decision to let it go.
2.   Accept what happened.
3.   Let go, when?
4.   Do not blame others.
5.   Focus on the present time and the joy in your life.
6.   Forgive them and yourself.

## Cultivate Empathy

Try to remember the other person's good qualities, assume that their motives were not meant to purposely cause you pain. Research has shown that empathy is associated with forgiveness and can make the process easier. Instead of seeing them as the "enemy," try to understand the factors that they were dealing with.

## Compassion

Compassion is the humane quality of understanding the suffering of others and wanting to do something about it. It is only natural that we wish to show compassion toward our peers. Compassion is a deep and personal emotion and is defined as the ability to understand the emotional state of another person.

There are many different ways to show compassion for others. The important thing is that it should come from your heart. Whether you are interacting with a friend, colleague, parents or family member, here are some ways you can demonstrate your compassion. "If you want others to be happy, practice compassion. If you want to be happy, practice compassion," says the Dalai Lama. According to the latest science, true happiness comes from practicing compassion. It is when we help our fellow man, when we feel connected to the world. When we give, expecting nothing in return, when we are kind, just to be kind, this is when life takes on meaning and purpose. Spreading joy throughout the world, we must practice compassion and kindness, which will open the door to the best of health benefits.

What works?

1. Start with yourself. Focus on your strength and positive qualities. Praise yourself for your successes and forgive yourself for your mistakes.
2. Communicate verbally. Make eye contact, keep your body toward the person speaking, and listen quietly.
3. Touch. A gentle touch goes a long way. To be sure that touch is welcome, ask first. Try, "Would you like a hug?" Gentle touch assists in balancing physical, mental, emotional, and spiritual well-being.
4. Encourage others. Positive reinforcement is always helpful to a person who is thinks they are stuck and will never get out of the circumstances they are in at that moment.
5. Express yourself. Match your facial expressions with your feelings to let another person know you understand what they are going through. A good laugh can be incredibly healing too.
6. Show kindness. Give your kindness away without expecting anything back. The world is made better through your kindness. Try smiling at a stranger today.

So many problems in our world come from a lack of compassion. Violence and hatred could be solved with a little compassion or a little understanding that we are all humans with strengths and weaknesses. For me, compassion and empathy go hand in hand. I challenge myself to be compassionate each and every day, whether that is with my clients or friends or my relatives. Kindness is expressed in ways big or small. It is the little things people remember the most. It may be just a kind word or a sincere compliment. Those people that work with serving others need to smile and say hello and wave to others. Starting today, treat everyone you meet as if they were going to be dead by midnight. Extend to them all the care, kindness, and understanding you can muster; and do it with no thought of any reward. Your life will never be the same again. This quote comes from Og Manino, author of *The Greatest Salesman in the World*.

## Friendliness

One of the most important human needs is connection with others. People want to be appreciated and respected, which is why there any many benefits of being friendly with people you meet. Being friendly will improve mental health issues. Friendly people are never alone. Everyone would like to have a kind, caring, humble individual as their companion. Having a friendly attitude will always benefit you in every phase of your life. Everyone will recognize and appreciate your friendly nature, and they will give you assistance in time of need.

How to be friendly

Recognize people for who they are. One of the interesting things about human perception is that we always see things from a specific point of view—our own. Recognizing someone else for who they are means finding the capacity to step outside ourselves. If we can find a way to see people for who they are—individuals with lives, hopes, dreams, struggles and victories—to see them as we often see ourselves, we can find more compassion, more friendliness toward them. You need to learn how to compliment people. One way you can learn to be friendlier is to compliment others. We shouldn't find it difficult to tell someone they did a good job or look good. We live in a world where we are bombarded by negativity. Try to compliment at least three people a day. Dealing with people is probably the biggest problem you will face, especially if you are in business. Develop a team spirit when working with others. Say things like, "Don't worry, I trust your judgment," or, "What else can I do to help?" or, "I just want you to know how much you mean to the team." Gratitude is another important thing with friendship. It brings compassion. Living gratefully makes us aware of beauty and kindness around us and makes us want to share blessings with others. You can say things like, "Thanks for always being willing to lend a hand," or, "Thank you for being so flexible," or even, "I could not have done it without you." Marcel Proust once said, "Let us be grateful to people who make us happy. They are the charming gardeners who make our souls blossom."

## The Spirituality of Pets

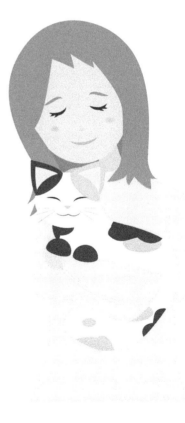

Animals play an essential part of the grand plan of life. They are like spiritual sponges, who absorb and uplift the love you give them. Today many pets have a job as therapy animals of the household. They might assist a member of the household physically or emotionally or to provide comfort to people. The human-animal body mind connection is a deeper assessment of the mental, emotional, physical, and spiritual connection between humans and animals. It often serves by reflecting back to us the lessons we are here to learn. Our animals know us better than almost any other being on the planet. They see what is in our minds. Their eyes see what is in our mind's eye. They feel what we feel and are often closer to our hearts than anyone else. For example, dogs are always communicating with us. By listening to our dogs, our lives can be turned into something incredible by just letting go of our desire to control them. Dogs are healers, no matter if they are therapy dogs, service dogs, or working dogs.

Same goes with cats. We tend to think of cats as cute little furry things and nothing more, often unaware of the fact that cats are some of the most powerful healers. Scientific studies have shown time and time again that cats are more than just great pets. They are extremely therapeutic and may actually be a good form of medicine for people suffering from a heart condition. Owning a cat can cut your risk of a heart attack. Many people have observed that a cat will come to help its owner when they are sick. Cats remove negative energy and restore body's ability to function fully again.

The more we open to the spiritual gifts our pets bring to us, the more they can share those gifts. Animals are a great blessing for people who do healing work. Healers love their talents and the joy those talents bring to others. They are like cleaning ladies who come into our consciousness and mop up the spills caused by the emotional turmoil of daily living. Studies have been done which show people who own pets will recover faster from an operation or that elderly people live longer and happier lives if they have a pet. Since animals help us transmute our unhappiness and negativity, pets help each one of us to become a better person.

# About the Author

Ramute Moye holds a doctorate of agricultural science, is an alternative medicine consultant, holistic energy healer, and integrative nutrition coach. She speaks three languages: Lithuanian, Russian, and English. She was born in Lithuania, a small country near the Baltic Sea. Her family had an extremely difficult time just hoping to survive World War II.

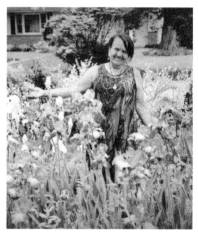

In 1941, during the Soviet occupation, most Lithuanian educated families and property owners were sent to Siberia. The people were packed into rail cars with locked doors and no windows. Many died along the way. At this time, Lithuania lost five hundred thousand people. When Nazi Germany declared war on the USSR, they occupied Lithuania, persecuting the Jews. By 1944, the Nazis were losing, which led to the return of the Soviets and even more brutality.

After World War II, Lithuania had even less educated people, with a majority that could neither read nor write. Ramute's parents were literate, but education was not held in high esteem. Rather, her family and most people lived a subsistence lifestyle raising animals and growing crops for food. Growing up under seemingly constant stress and often not having enough food, she, like many children, was often sick. Many of her fellow Lithuanian children died. Ramute became paralyzed at the age of five on the left side of body, and at age ten, she contracted tuberculosis. To complicate the matters further, at age twelve, she was diagnosed with a gallbladder infection and was prescribed a list of medications which led to numerous side effects. During this time of tribulation, she continued to believe that there surely is a better way to live and dreamed of a better life.

At the age of fourteen, she left home and started living at an agriculture high school for the next few years. It was there that she earned her first diploma of agricultural sciences and started her work as an agronomist. She resumed her graduate studies at the University of Agriculture of Lithuania and was awarded her master's degree in agriculture and continued to complete a PhD in agriculture science.

For the next twenty years, she worked as manager of agriculture for a county in Lithuania. She was in charge of producing increasing higher yields for forty-nine farms within the county. Following the common beliefs of the day, she recommended the use of pesticides, chemicals, and fertilizers, achieving higher yields. She didn't connect the chemicals to her feeling tired and sick so much of the time. Until one day, Ramute heard about organic farming techniques. She applied to study organic farming in the United States. After learning about organic farming in the US, she returned to the Institute of Horticulture in Lithuania. There she refined her skills and wrote a book *Biohumus and Organic Farming* (2006), implemented the organic farming within her county, and gave many speeches extolling the virtues of organic gardening.

In addition to becoming an organic gardener, she became interested in holistic healing, which led her to the world of alternative medicine, as well as yoga and meditation. She enrolled in the Integrative Nutrition Health Coach program in 2017 graduating in 2018. She is a public speaker, co-leader at her house of worship. She belongs to two garden clubs and is very active in her community.

Ramute enriched her life by becoming an organic gardener. For the last twenty years, she has practiced holistic healing, utilizing homemade remedies, yoga, and meditation rather than taking pharmaceuticals. She looks and feels much healthier than most people her age. She has been trained by world renowned coach Mary Morrissey, and worldwide energy healer Deborah King. At the Institute of Integrative Nutrition, she learned how important it is to have healthy relationships, to have a positive work-life balance, and to live in the present.

*This book will guide you on making the right choice in the foods you eat, loving yourself and others, and practicing a spiritually enlightened lifestyle. Ramute's dream is to share these life lessons with you so you could be healthy, happy, and live your life to the fullest!*

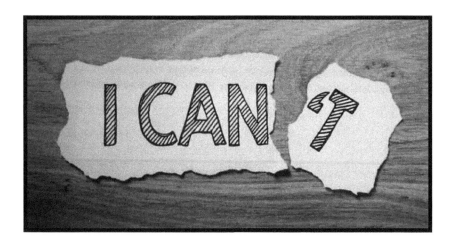

Ingram Content Group UK Ltd.
Milton Keynes UK
UKHW022302030423
419516UK00010B/117